GIVING BIRTH CAN BE THE MOST
JOYOUS AND FULFILLING EXPERIENCE
YOU HAVE EVER KNOWN.

IF YOU LET IT BE.

This book will show you how to exercise your body.

It will show you how to relax your body.

It will show you how to give your body the help
it needs when you need it the most—

THE COMPLETE PREGNANCY
EXERCISE PROGRAM

ABOUT THE AUTHOR:

DIANA SIMKIN has a master's degree in dance
education from New York University and has been
teaching pregnancy exercise classes since 1974.
She is currently the Exercise Director at the
Elisabeth Bing Center for Parents in New York City
and is an instructor of the Lamaze technique
of childbirth.

THE COMPLETE PREGNANCY EXERCISE PROGRAM

By Diana Simkin

With a Foreword by Elisabeth Bing

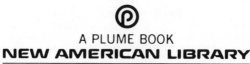

A PLUME BOOK

NEW AMERICAN LIBRARY

TIMES MIRROR

NEW YORK, LONDON AND SCARBOROUGH, ONTARIO

To all my students

NAL BOOKS ARE AVAILABLE AT QUANTITY DISCOUNTS WHEN USED TO
PROMOTE PRODUCTS OR SERVICES. FOR INFORMATION PLEASE WRITE TO
PREMIUM MARKETING DIVISION, THE NEW AMERICAN LIBRARY, INC.,
1633 BROADWAY, NEW YORK, NEW YORK 10019.

Library of Congress Cataloging in Publication Data

Simkin, Diana.
The complete pregnancy exercise program.

1. Pregnancy.   2. Prenatal care.   3. Postnatal
care.   4. Exercise for women.   I. Title.
RG558.7.S58   1980   618.2′4   80-36712
ISBN 0-452-25243-1

PLUME TRADEMARK REG. PAT. U.S. OFF. AND FOREIGN COUNTRIES
REGISTERED TRADEMARK—MARCA REGISTRADA
HECHO EN WESTFORD, MASS., U.S.A.

SIGNET, SIGNET CLASSICS, MENTOR, PLUME, MERIDIAN, and
NAL BOOKS are published in the United States by The New American
Library, 1633 Broadway, New York, New York 10019, in Canada by
The New American Library of Canada Limited, 81 Mack Avenue,
Scarborough, Ontario M1L 1M8, in the United Kingdom by The New
English Library Limited, Barnard's Inn, Holborn,
London, EC1N 2JR England.

First Printing, October, 1980

2   3   4   5   6   7   8   9

PRINTED IN THE UNITED STATES OF AMERICA

With special thanks to my husband, David Kritchman, for his unending patience; to Amanda Kreglow for photographing the prenatal exercises and to Gayle Pines Driver for being my prenatal model; to Richard Brummett for photographing the postnatal exercises and to Ginger Novak for doing the makeup; to Elisabeth Bing for her kindness and generosity over the years in sharing her knowledge with me; to my teacher, Kathy Grant, from whom I've learned so much; to my editor, Ann Watson, for her constant and steady support; and especially to all my students, past and present, who have made my work so interesting and rewarding.

CONTENTS

FOREWORD

We live in an interesting and strange time. On one hand, advanced technology affects every part of our lives, offering great advances for many, and yet on the other, industrial waste pollutes our cities, our countryside, even our food. Ironically, environmental deterioration makes us more and more aware of the needs of a healthy body, which are often not met by desk jobs and processed foods. Many of us try to eat nourishing foods to control our cholesterol levels, diet to keep slim, and exercise to keep fit.

This understandable concern for good health strongly affects the pregnant woman, who wishes to enjoy her body throughout her pregnancy but is aware that until recently society considered women to be unusually vulnerable at this time. Of course, not all women were actually privileged to lead sedentary lives when they were expecting a baby. There have always been young mothers who worked hard physically and still gave birth to healthy babies. In fact, we know that women who had to work for their livelihood in the fields seemed to have easier births. Perhaps it is this knowledge, combined with improved medical care and the increased awareness of the importance of a fit body, which encourages modern women to feel confident about exercising their bodies during pregnancy.

With our new perception of the benefits of exercise, today's young women feel almost guilty when they restrict their movements the moment they are pregnant. Yet, decades of cultural conditioning which insisted on non-movement cannot always be overcome even today, and a pregnant woman may find herself puzzled as to how to keep her changing body strong and well-exercised.

The Complete Pregnancy Exercise Program is therefore especially welcome, as Diana Simkin, an experienced pregnancy exercise teacher, offers the pregnant woman not only a variety of complete exercise routines but also advice on how to exercise safely and how to take care of herself during pregnancy. Her philosophy is that pregnancy is not an illness women have to be treated for, but rather a healthy physiological state.

This book gives all pregnant women a healthy and sensible approach to exercise during the nine months of pregnancy and after, and above all, it provides a wonderfully practical routine for daily exercising. I have myself participated in the classes the author holds, and I know that her routines exercise the entire body, with special emphasis on those muscles which are most used during pregnancy and those muscles which will be used in labor. The exercises strengthen and stretch the muscles, encourage good posture and mobility, and teach a woman to move as gracefully as possible.

Diana does not neglect the postpartum period. Her suggestions and routines for after the baby is born have been carefully designed and clearly explained so that each woman can enjoy the return of her prenatal body. I have long advocated healthy and natural movement during pregnancy, and I hope that more and more young mothers will discover the great benefits of exercises during and after pregnancy through this excellently researched book.

Elisabeth Bing
Clinical Assistant Professor,
Department of Obstetrics and Gynecology
New York Medical College

INTRODUCTION

You may have exercised regularly for the past five years or you may never have exercised at all, but now that you are pregnant you probably have a number of questions about what kind of exercise is safe. Pregnancy is a healthy state rather than the delicate condition it was once thought to be. Today, women are encouraged to continue their daily routines, including sports, work, and hobbies, and regular exercise is recognized as a major factor in contributing toward a healthy and more comfortable pregnancy.

Unless your doctor has cautioned you against strenuous exertions because of a specific medical problem such as toxemia or high blood pressure, you can do anything when you are pregnant that you could do before, for as long as you feel like it. You can stretch your arms above your head, take baths, ride your bike, sleep on your stomach, lift and hold your older child, exercise, and do all those other things you normally include in your busy daily life.

Nature has seen to it that your baby is extremely well protected, not only by the bony spine and pelvis and by layers of muscle and tissue, but also by the soft cushion of amniotic fluid that surrounds it. Exercising and other strenuous activities will not hurt the fetus, hurt you, cause your membranes to rupture, or start labor. Many women whose due dates have come and gone have continued to come to my exercise classes in the hope that labor would be triggered. It never is. Labor will begin when it's time, and not before.

Exercise is extremely important. It will keep you feeling healthy and energetic during your pregnancy, help you to carry your baby with ease and grace, help prepare you for the physical work of giving birth to your baby, and ease and hasten your postpartum recovery. Exercise will also help you to keep in touch with your changing body and give you a more positive mental outlook.

The exercises in this book are the same ones I teach in my prenatal and postnatal exercise classes. You can do them safely at home in conjunction with your regular fitness program, or to replace it. These exercises are also suitable even if you have never exercised before. Begin the prenatal exercises as early in your pregnancy as you can, and continue doing them for as long as you like. There is no point at which you should stop, or at which you are too pregnant to exercise unless a specific medical problem arises. Start the postnatal exercises as soon as you have your doctor's or midwife's go-ahead (usually about four weeks after birth), and again, continue for as long as you like, even into your next pregnancy.

This book discusses not only which exercises to do during pregnancy and after, but also the whys, hows, and feelings associated with each exercise. It's one thing to copy a movement from a book and another thing to understand why you're doing it, how to execute it correctly, and how it should feel. The descriptions and suggestions for each exercise will help you to perform the movements correctly so that you will derive the maximum benefit from them. If you follow the instructions, you'll learn to do the exercises in a way that makes inner physical sense, using the correct muscles rather than just copying the superficial shape of a movement from a picture on a page.

The exercises that follow have been developed for the special needs of pregnancy and after. They are almost all adaptations of dance and yoga movement phrases I've learned, performed, and taught over the years. If the exercises are done properly they should make you feel relaxed and refreshed, and give you confidence in your body and a sense of health and well-being.

The pregnancy exercises will keep you feeling fit; the postpartum exercises will get your body back into shape and keep it that way. Feel free to continue to use these exercises for as long as you like, for good health in years to come.

I WHY EXERCISE?

During pregnancy, the abdominal muscles and tissues stretch to accommodate a uterus that will expand to about twenty times its usual size. The intestines are displaced up and to the back as the baby grows. The diaphragm is pressed upward and has less mobility, but the ribs expand to make up for this loss of space. Blood plasma volume increases by about 40 percent and the heart not only pumps more blood but does it faster than normally, increasing the amount of blood it pumps per minute by thirty to forty percent. Then, there are all the hormonal changes as well.

Even though your body is capable of adapting naturally to the changes it will be undergoing during your pregnancy, exercise will help you to cope with these changes more easily.

For one thing, exercise will improve your blood circulation so that you can avoid or ease such common pregnancy problems as varicose veins, swollen hands and feet, and leg cramps (see Chapter VI).

Exercise will also help keep your pelvic, spinal, and abdominal muscles toned and strong and therefore better able to support the added weight of the uterus and baby. Lower back pain, once thought to be an unavoidable part of pregnancy, can be relieved if not completely alleviated through exercise and good postural habits. (see posture pg. 19) Having good support from below will take the strain off your back and enable you to carry your baby more easily and gracefully.

Exercise will help prepare your body for the work of labor and delivery. There's a reason why the process of childbirth is called labor—it's hard work! And because it's physical work, your body needs to be in good condition.

If you exercise regularly, you will have the strength and stamina needed for childbirth. You will have confidence in your body and you'll cope more easily with the physical and mental stress of labor. During the first stage you'll be able to relax and breathe with each contraction. During the delivery, you'll know where and how to push the baby out. If your abdominal muscles are strong, your delivery will be easier and probably take less time, and the likelihood of needing a forceps delivery will be decreased.

During labor you will want to be able to conserve energy as much as possible. If, as your uterus contracts you tense your whole body with it (a very natural response if it hurts), you will create a lot of muscular tension. This tension will tire you (working muscles require energy while resting ones do not), make you even more uncomfortable during your labor, and make it more difficult for your cervix to dilate (open) smoothly. If, through exercise, you can learn to use only those muscles that you need and consciously relax the ones you don't, you will be much better equipped to handle your labor.

More than ever, you need the psychological ego boost that exercise will give you. When you're feeling good about yourself mentally, it will be reflected in your physical appearance. Your posture will improve, you'll walk taller and hold your head higher. My students are always being told how good they look (often with a note of surprise, as if looking pregnant and looking good were mutually exclusive)! Really, it's very simple. They look good because they feel good.

If you have exercised throughout your pregnancy, your postpartum recovery will be faster and easier. Women who are in poor physical condition often complain of soreness and exhaustion the day following birth. This does not have to happen to you. The only discomfort my students usually experience is around the epistiotomy (small incision many women have to ease and speed the birth of the baby), and even this can be lessened by doing the pelvic floor exercises described on pages 21-23.

One of the most obvious rewards of exercising will be the speed with which you will return to your prepregnancy shape (or better) since your muscles will respond quickly to postpartum exercise. You will also have maintained the internal structural support in the abdomen and pelvic floor necessary for good health.

Exercising will give your body strength, muscle tone, and flexibility. It will help you to develop new powers of concentration and relaxation and to become aware of how to use your muscles most effectively. Breathing while you exercise will enable you to relax while you stretch and to keep your body well oxygenated as you work. These abilities will also help you during childbirth.

By exercising just fifteen or twenty minutes a day, you will be more likely to have a healthy, problem-free pregnancy, carry your baby easily and gracefully, enjoy the experience of your pregnant body, and be well equipped (with the added help of prepared childbirth classes) to handle your labor and delivery. Your body will recover quickly and with a minimum of discomfort.

II ESTABLISHING·THE EXERCISE HABIT

One needs discipline to exercise at home, for there is always the temptation to put exercising aside for other chores. The solution is to accept the importance of including exercise as an integral part of your daily routine, rather than as a luxury to be enjoyed whenever it can be worked into your busy schedule. To be most effective, it should be high on your list of priorities. There can't be any choice about whether to exercise today or tomorrow, in the morning or later in the day. It should be made a firm part of your schedule, a part that doesn't get slept through, rearranged, postponed, or canceled "just for today."

Time

Choose a time that is best for you, when you will be undisturbed. If you are an early riser, try to arrange your morning to accommodate fifteen to twenty minutes of exercise. Some good stretching followed by a shower will energize you for the day ahead. If, however, you don't even feel alive, much less like exercising, when you rise in the morning, schedule a time later in the day, perhaps while your older child is napping or at school, or early in the evening when you come home from work. Your husband may even want to join you—these exercises are just as beneficial for him. You may at first think you feel too tired, but if you discipline yourself to just change your clothes and start, you'll find that by the end of your routine you'll feel relaxed and refreshed.

Place

Clear a space in your home (or office, if you have one) with enough room to move comfortably without kicking your bed, desk, or coffee table each time you stretch your foot. If your space is too confining, or you're worried about knocking something over, you will be tense and hesitant about stretching fully. Very often, just moving a chair or two out of the way is all that's required. A carpeted room is best, but a blanket, towel, or exercise mat underneath to soften the floor will do just as well.

If you can, exercise where you can see yourself in a mirror. You shouldn't be looking at it all the time, but it can be very useful in helping you make corrections, just the way a dancer uses the mirror in a dance class. For example, you may be doing the Graham Stretch, or the Table Top I and think your back is straight. If you check yourself in the mirror you will probably find that improvements can be made.

The room you use should be warm, not cool. Exercises warm up the muscles in the body to make them more limber, so exercising in a cold room only defeats the purpose. The space should also be well ventilated, but you should never be in the direct line of a draft from fans, windows, or air-conditioners. Cold air hitting warm muscles causes them to contract or tighten, which in turn can cause cramping or even muscle spasms.

Eating

Don't eat just before exercising. During pregnancy the baby takes up precious room usually occupied by the stomach and intestines, and most women find they are uncomfortable lying on the floor if they've just eaten. Even if you are not pregnant, eating before exercising can be uncomfortable. If you're hungry or feel you need to eat something, try having some juice or some crackers to tide you over until you can sit down to a meal.

Clothing

Wear whatever feels comfortable. Shorts and a T-shirt, leotards and tights, or sweat pants and a top are all loose and unconfining. One woman I know wore her husband's old boxer shorts (the elastic had stretched) and a T-shirt. Another woman wore one-piece long underwear like a union suit. None of these were the latest in exercise attire, but they did the trick nonetheless.

Music

Put on a record or play the radio while you exercise. A record album lasts just about the right amount of time (although exercising longer is certainly fine, too) and it will help to put you in the mood to move. Play anything that you like to listen to and let the music keep you company while you move.

III YOUR EXERCISE PROGRAM

You may begin the exercises in this book at any time during your pregnancy or after, but remember, the earlier you start the sooner you will begin to benefit. Women have joined my prenatal exercise classes anywhere from the third to the ninth month of their pregnancies, and my postnatal exercise classes from two weeks to seven months after giving birth. It will do you good whenever you start, but sooner *is* better, since the earlier you start, the more time you will have to learn the exercises, establish the exercise habit and get your body into condition.

You should be able to continue the prenatal exercises until the day you deliver. The specific exercises you choose may change as your belly gets larger and heavier, but it's important to continue, not only because it will make you feel better, but also because it will help you maintain your strength and stamina. Toward the end of your pregnancy you will probably prefer the sitting exercises to the ones on your back. If this happens, adjust your routine accordingly. You may also prefer to exercise more slowly or to perform the movements at a more relaxed pace. However, unless there's a medical contraindication such as premature labor or hypertension, there's really no reason for you to stop.

Ideally, you should exercise at least fifteen to twenty minutes every day. If this is impossible (although it shouldn't be if you are truly committed), exercise at least three times each week. Regular, frequent exercise will result in obvious improvements in strength, relaxation, and flexibility. The exercises will become more familiar more quickly and you'll notice that they'll become easier to do. Exercise once or twice a week will still be better than nothing, but you are doing yourself a disservice. Irregular, infrequent exercise is like treading water—you're doing something, but it won't really get you anywhere.

HOW TO USE THIS BOOK

This book contains twenty-four prenatal and twenty-four postnatal exercises which have been divided into a total of six exercise programs of eight exercises each. Each program is a complete fifteen-minute exercise routine.

I have also included six standing exercises, three for pregnancy and three for after, which appear at the end of each exercise chapter. They get you up off the floor and allow you to work your entire body in a freer, more coordinated way than you do in the other exercises. They are included as optional movements because they will add more time to your daily routine. However, I usually end my classes standing and so I have included them for you to try if you like. You may want to start with these exercises and then proceed to the ones on the floor; either method is fine, or you can skip the standing exercises altogether.

Before starting, look over the exercises in the program you'll be doing. Read the instructions carefully and look closely at the pictures. Once you have read the program yourself, try to have your husband or a friend read the instructions aloud, repeating the suggestions and corrections while you do the exercises, and checking to see that what you are doing corresponds to the photographs. You may even get some company if your helper decides to join you. If you cannot find a reader, keep the book handy so that you can consult it as needed. Be patient; it will take time before you will begin to feel comfortable with each set of exercises. Try to memorize each routine as you perform it, and concentrate on developing a sense of rhythm to the movements so that you will be able to move smoothly from one exercise to the next.

When you begin these exercises, do not worry about following the specific breathing instructions. Learn the movements first, and make sure that you do not hold your breath as you move. Once you feel comfortable with the exercises, try to breathe as recommended. After a while, you will find that the breathing becomes an integral part of the exercises, helping you to do them more easily. A detailed discussion of how to breathe correctly can be found on pages 13-14.

Spend a minimum of three to four weeks learning each routine in the order in which they are presented so that after nine to twelve weeks you will have mastered either all the prenatal or all the postnatal exercises.

As previously noted, each routine should take from fifteen to twenty minutes to complete. If you find that you finish in less than fifteen minutes, you are rushing through the exercises and you should slow down. If it takes you longer, you are probably either doing each exercise too many times or resting too long between exercises. Resting between exercises for more than a few moments will defeat the warming-up process, and prevent you from developing stamina.

Exercise carefully! A woman's body changes during pregnancy, and even familiar exercises can feel unfamiliar. Go slowly at first until you begin to feel comfortable with the exercises. It's not how rapidly you can finish that counts, but how well the movements are executed while you work. If you are short on exercise time one day, simply do fewer exercises rather than rushing through your entire routine double time.

Before you start to exercise, take a few moments to prepare yourself. Get into position for your first exercise, close your eyes, and take three slow deep breaths. Concentrate on what you are doing now, not what you were doing or thinking about before you started or what you will be doing after you finish. Begin when you are ready. Move gently through the first exercise of your routine to allow your body to warm up gradually. In this way you will be exercising with conscious thought and minimizing the possibility of injury.

Keep in mind that the same exercises will feel different on different days. Our bodies change and react from day to day (and even hour to hour) to differences in the weather, our mood, the amount of sleep we have had and other factors. One day you may feel fabulously limber and the next day tight and inflexible. If you do feel tight or tired one day, don't force yourself to accomplish what you did the day before. Circumstances are different. Take each day and each exercise session one at a time and enjoy your progress as it occurs over the course of weeks rather than from one day to the next.

Do not be concerned if you cannot perform a given exercise as gracefully as the models seem to in the photographs. These are presented as an ideal to be worked toward rather than what should or can be immediately copied. The exercises may be difficult at first, but with practice and repetition, you will find that they will become consistently easier as you become stronger and your muscles become more toned and flexible.

CREATING YOUR OWN EXERCISE PROGRAM

Should you find that you grow attached to a single routine, feel free to continue the exercises in that program. You do not have to change routines. However, many women like to change the exercises they do for variety's sake so that exercising doesn't become "routine" or boring; many prefer different exercises as their pregnancies progress. In this case, you can design your own program, using your favorite exercises to develop the one that is the best for you.

Never force yourself to do an exercise just because you think it is good for you. I have found that women (myself included) who dislike a particular exercise "tune out" mentally while doing it and therefore do not benefit from it. Simply replace it with a related exercise that you do like and that you will do correctly.

Keep in mind that every exercise has its benefits whether it is a simple Pelvic Tilt or Single Leg Slide or a more complicated Coccyx Balance. Do not be misled into thinking that the best exercises are the most difficult ones, or that the best routines have the most strenuous and impressive-looking movements. This is a common misconception and often interferes with your ability to exercise effectively.

Each program in this book includes both stretching and strengthening exercises. Both are equally important to a well-rounded program. Each also includes exercises for the hips, waist, abdomen, upper body, back, legs and feet. If you decide to design your own program make sure that it also includes exercises for every body part. In this way, you will be working toward your goal of being toned and strong, yet maintaining and increasing your flexibility and range of motion. Use the charts at the end of this chapter to help you.

BREATHING

Pay close attention to your breathing while you exercise. Proper breathing keeps your muscles well oxygenated and actively helps you while you work. It's all too easy to stop breathing for short periods of time or to breathe shallowly while concentrating on an exercise. Try instead to think about breathing smoothly and rhythmically and you will find that the movements will be more easily and gracefully performed. Tension will be released, not created.

Learning to breathe properly while you exercise will also help you in labor. Labor involves muscular work just like exercising, so it follows that if you've been using the breathing to help you while you exercise, you can also use it to help you during a labor contraction. You will keep your baby well oxygenated, your body will be better able to metabolize the waste products produced by working muscles, and you will get less tired.

Our breathing is intimately connected with our physical and emotional states. We breathe more rapidly after strenuous physical exertions such as running up a flight of stairs or moving heavy furniture. It can also speed up or stop completely under emotional stress when we're angry, surprised, or upset ("It so surprised me, it took my breath away"). On the other hand, our breathing tends to be quiet and rhythmical during dreamless sleep or when we're feeling calm and relaxed.

This interrelatonship can be used to our advantage—consciously slowing down our breathing when we're upset can enable us to handle a situation more rationally and effectively. That old advice when we're upset or nervous to "Stop and take three deep breaths," works.

This is one of the reasons many prepared childbirth techniques teach specific breathing patterns. In labor (and at other stressful times) the tendency is often to either hold one's breath or breathe very rapidly, neither of which is good for you or the baby, serving only to create more tension and anxiety. If you've practiced the exercises with an awareness of your breathing, you will be better able to breathe calmly and rhythmically during your labor or at other times and thereby lessen your discomfort.

You'll find specific breathing instructions for most of the exercises in this book. In the beginning, while you are first learning the exercises, concentrate on what the movements are and think only about breathing evenly. Keep checking yourself while you exercise to make sure you're not holding your breath.

Once the movements are familiar, try the specific breathing pattern in the instructions. You'll discover that the suggestions make physical sense and have a logic to them. For example, legs usually stretch away from the body during exhalations and toward the body during inhalations (Leg Stretches I, Single Leg Slide, Leg Stretches Opening Side). You'll almost always use your abdominal muscles during the exhalations and relax your abdomen during the inhalations. The most difficult movements are performed while you breathe out to help you to use your abdominal muscles more strongly, while the easier movements occur as you relax and breathe in.

If a suggested breathing pattern doesn't work for you, experiment with others until you find a better pattern. For example, in the Back Massage (page 34) you may want to inhale to start, exhale on the way up, inhale at the top, and exhale on the way down. Or you may want to inhale all the way up and exhale all the way down. If the tempo at which you're exercising is different from mine, you will probably have to change the breathing pattern from the one presented. That's fine. What's important is that you find what works for you.

Let your breathing help you. You'll find yourself with an invaluable tool.

HELPFUL HINTS FOR EXERCISING

The following suggestions will help you to move correctly. Although they are apparently simple and straightforward, most people are not aware of these principles of movement. If you apply them while you exercise, you will move more easily and effectively.

• Whenever you move from a bent-knee position to a straight leg, such as in the Single Leg Slide, and all the Leg Stretches, do not think of straightening your knee. It seems that whenever there is concentration on the knee itself, there follows a sharpness of movement which can strain, or cause damage to the knee. Instead, try to think of lengthening the muscles in the back of your entire leg, stretching it gently in one smooth motion as if it were underwater.

• Use *the principle of opposition* whenever possible. Moving is physical, and one of the laws of physics is that for every action, there is an equal and opposite reaction. Applied to movement, this means that whatever muscles aren't working to move a body part are working to hold the rest of the body steady. You are never using just one body part. In fact, the muscles in the nonmoving parts of the body are usually the ones that work the hardest. For example, in the Leg Stretches Opening Side (page 66), it's easy to open your leg to the side, but it's difficult to do so while still keeping your lower back, both hips, and both shoulders flat on the floor at the same time. The leg is moving to the side, but your abdominal muscles, the muscles in your back, and others all work to make it possible.

Opposition can also be used to obtain a deeper and fuller stretch, such as in doing the Head Circles (page 38). Drop your head to your right side, so your right ear faces your right shoulder. What do you feel? Now leave your head where it is and pull your left shoulder down, away from your head. Do you feel how the opposition of the two body parts—your head and your shoulder—can create a stronger stretch?

If you are aware of this movement principle, you will discover many exercises to which it can be applied. You will be able to move correctly, stretch the muscles in your body more fully and deeply, and exercise with a more complete awareness of what you are doing.

• In the instructions to many of the sitting exercises, I mention the *"sit bones."* Technically, they are called the ischial tuberosities and are the bottom tips of the part of the pelvis called the ischium. Sit on a hard surface. Rock your buttocks from side to side. Do you feel two bones? Now sit still with your hips evenly placed over your sit bones, your ribs evenly over your hips, your spine long and straight, and your head and neck centered over your ribs and shoulders. Think of a plumb line through your body from the top of your head down through the center of your body and out between your sit bones to the floor. This is your *center position.*

When I exercise, I use these sit bones as a bony landmark. They tell me if I am sitting with my weight evenly balanced or centered over my pelvis. If I can feel one side more than the other, I know that I must be leaning to that side and can correct myself. In this way, I don't need a mirror to tell me if I'm straight.

Try to be aware of these bones when you do any of the sitting exercises, such as the Side Stretches, Body Circles, or the Leg Stretch With Twist. Every time you return to center from a forward or side position, balance your body right on top of these bones.

The Prenatal Exercises

Abdomen

Back Massage
Leg Stretches I
Leg Stretches Opening Side
Open Pelvic Tilt
Pelvic Tilt
Side Knee Drops
Side Leg Lifting
Single Leg Slide
Sitting Pelvic Tilt
V-Stretch

Back

Arm Circles
Back Massage
Body Circles
Body Twist
Open Pelvic Tilt
Pelvic Tilt
Side Knee Drops
Sitting Pelvic Tilt
Sitting Side Stretches

Upper Body/Arms

Arm Circles
Body Circles
Body Twist
Head Circles
Sitting Side Stretches

Legs/Feet

Ankle Circles
Back Massage
Footwork
Hamstring Stretch
Leg Stretches I
Leg Stretches Opening Side
Side Leg Lifting
Side Leg Stretches
Single Leg Slide
Thigh Stretch
V-Stretch

Hips/Waist

Body Circles
Body Twist
Side Knee Drops
Side Leg Lifting
Side Press
Sitting Side Stretches
Thigh Stretch

Entire Body

Graham Stretch
Leg Stretch with Twist
Pliés/Relevés
Side Stretch in Stride
Standing Side Stretch I
Table Top I

The Postnatal Exercises

Abdomen

Coccyx Balance
Double Leg Slide
Grace
Knee Changes
Leg Circles
Leg Crossovers
Leg Lowering
Leg Stretches II
Reverse Sit-Ups
Side Knee Rolling
Sitting Leg Slide

Back

Back Massage With Leg Stretch
Full Body Circles With Arms
Coccyx Balance
Hip Circles
Knee Changes
Knee Cross
Shoulder Stretch
Shoulder Circles
Side Knee Rolling
Sitting Leg Slide
Snow Angels

Upper Body/Arms

Chest Lift
Full Body Circles With Arms
Grace
Knee Cross
Shoulder Circles
Shoulder Stretch

Side Knee Rolling
Snow Angels

Legs/Feet

Back Massage With Leg Stretch
Double Leg Lifting
Full Body Circles With Arms
Hip Circles
Knee Changes
Leg Circles
Leg Crossovers
Leg Stretches II
Side Thighs
Sitting Hamstring Stretch

Hips/Waist

Back Massage With Leg Stretch
Body Circles with Arms
Double Leg Lifting
Grace
Hip Circles
Knee Cross
Leg Crossovers
Side Knee Rolling

Entire Body

Chest Lift
Full Circles in Stride
Pliés/Relevés II
Shoulder Stand
Standing Side Stretch II
Table Top II

IV MOVING THROUGH YOUR DAY

POSTURE

You may exercise daily, but if your standing posture is poor or if you slump when you sit, you are undoing much of the good you do by exercising. Good posture not only makes you look and feel better, it also makes it easier to carry the baby both during pregnancy and after, gives you more internal room for your baby so it's easier to breathe, takes the strain off the lower back and pelvic muscles, and helps to keep the abdominal muscles toned.

The weight of a nonpregnant woman's body is centered in the middle of her pelvis. During pregnancy, however, the center shifts forward with the weight of the baby. Most women either give in to this weight by slumping forward or counter-balance this forward weight by leaning back with the upper body (increasing the curve in the lower back) and shifting their weight into their heels.

To determine whether this is happening to you, stand sideways to a full-length mirror and take a look at your posture. Are your shoulders drooping? Is there a deep hollow in your lower spine? If so, pull your abdominal muscles up and in and grow taller by lengthening your ribs away from your waist. Let your arms and head feel light and let your shoulders, spine, and buttocks relax.

Never squeeze your buttocks to tuck your hips forward. This is not the way to straighten the curve in your lower back. I know many books and magazine articles recommend it, but it is absolutely wrong. It will affect the surface look of your posture, but it's only a cosmetic change pasted to the outside of your body. Inside, it creates more tension in the muscles of the lower back and encourages the abdominal muscles to weaken. Besides, how can you walk with your buttocks squeezed?

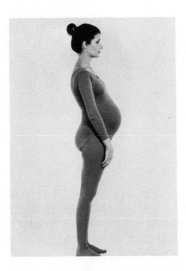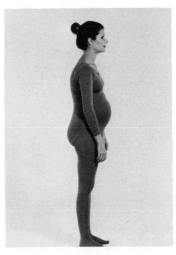

For good posture whether you are standing or sitting, lift your ribs up and away from your waist, tighten the abdominal muscles, and let your back and buttocks relax. Feel that your spine is very long. If you are standing you will notice that the weight of your body is placed more toward your toes than your heels. There will also still be a slight curve in your lower spine. This is correct. If you are sitting, your back will be straight. If you check the mirror again you will see that your posture is now quite beautiful.

It will feel good to stand or sit correctly, but it will take a lot of active work before it also feels natural. New habits aren't always easy to establish, but the effort will be well worthwhile.

Until this new correct posture becomes second nature, check yourself around the house when you pass a mirror and in store windows as you walk by. Also, enlist the aid of your husband or a co-worker and ask him or her to gently remind you to stand or sit tall when you forget.

Wearing flat or low-heeled shoes will also help your posture. High heels are fashionable, but they are terrible for your back since they shift the weight of your body forward, out of its natural alignment. The curve in your lower spine is accentuated, the backs of your calves tighten, and adjustments are made throughout the entire

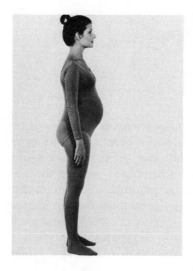

body to help you balance. During pregnancy, your weight is already forward so your body has to adjust even more. Lower shoes may not be stylish, but they will be comfortable and better for you.

THE PELVIC FLOOR

The pelvic floor is a very important set of muscles because it helps to support all the pelvic organs—including the bladder, rectum, vagina, and uterus. I like to imagine that it's like a muscular hammock slung from the pubic bone in front to the lower spine in back.

Technically, it's called the pubo-coccygeal muscle and it wraps itself around the urethra, vagina, and anus in a figure-eight-type pattern.

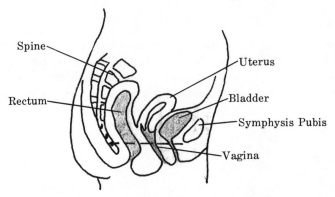

The pelvic floor helps to support all the pelvic contents.

The pelvic floor should be consciously exercised throughout one's lifetime, but it is usually not brought to a woman's attention until pregnancy. That's because during this time, the pelvic floor assumes an even greater importance—that of helping to support the added weight of the growing uterus and baby, placenta, and amniotic fluid. If these muscles are weak, the ability to support the pelvic organs will be impaired and may, after a period of time, result in poor bladder or rectal control, loss of tone in the vaginal walls which will decrease sexual pleasure during intercourse, or a uterine prolapse which will require surgical correction.

If, on the other hand, these muscles are kept in good tone by exercising them daily, they will be able to support the added weight of pregnancy, relax and stretch during labor and delivery, and return to good tone afterward. Prevention is the best and cheapest approach to health care. Exercise is free and painless—operations are not!

Isolating and exercising the pelvic floor can be accomplished in many different ways. One of the easiest ways is to practice when you urinate. Each time you go to the bathroom (and during pregnancy that's usually quite often), stop the flow of urine once or twice. It may be difficult at first, but you'll be amazed at how quickly you will improve. Another way is to try to feel that you can lift and tighten the pelvic hammock from the front to the back, squeezing the urethra (as you did to stop the flow of urine), the vaginal muscles, and then the rectal sphincter. Hold everything tightly (except your breath) for about five seconds, then *gently* release the muscles and feel them relax. Repeat the tightening and letting go twice more. These muscles cannot be completely separated, but you will with practice be able to feel a ripple effect as you tighten and then relax these muscles.

A pleasant and rewarding way to exercise the pelvic floor is by turning it into a "sexercise." During intercourse, squeeze your partner's penis by contracting the vaginal muscles. Let him tell you whether you've found the correct muscles. Again, it may be difficult to find the correct muscles at first, but it can be fun trying. And remember, practice makes perfect!

Practice while doing your regular exercise routine, so that each time you tighten your abdomen, you tighten your pelvic floor, too. Use both sets of muscles as you do the Pelvic Tilts (both lying on the floor and sitting up), Back Massage, Knee Drops, and the Pliés and Relevés. You will find that including the pelvic floor muscles in this way will not only keep your muscles toned, but will also make the exercises easier to do.

Obviously, the pelvic floor exercises can be done in many different ways at many different times. The exercises are invisible, so you can do them waiting for a bus or subway or for a light to change from red to green, while standing in line at the grocery store or bank, or while reading, washing dishes, or watching television. It's really only a matter of remembering. For optimum results, the pelvic floor should be exercised at least twenty to thirty times a day. That may sound like a lot, but it's easily accomplished once you've established the habit. And it's a good habit to maintain not only during your pregnancy, but from now on.

RELAXATION

I often like to begin or end my exercise classes with a five-to-ten-minute period of deep breathing and relaxation. It tends to refocus everyone's physical and mental energies from the concerns of their day to themselves and the class at hand or to refresh everyone after working hard in class.

It's often difficult to relax. Stuck in a traffic jam we tell ourselves that worrying won't get us to our appointments any faster, and so we may as well "just relax." At times like these, it's easier said than done. In fact, because most of us don't do it very often, we get out of practice. We forget *how* to relax.

In labor, it's very much the same. Being tense or anxious won't bring the baby any faster and may, in fact, have the opposite effect. Tensing the body during a contraction (1) will make your body have to work harder since more muscles are activated, (2) may increase your discomfort as you focus on your pain, and (3) will make it more difficult for your cervix to efface and dilate (thin and open). Therefore, the better you are at being able to relax, the more you ease the way for the physical changes of labor to occur and the easier it will be for you.

Being able to relax will also help you at other times. We all get tired or irritable if we haven't had enough sleep, if we're hungry, or if things just haven't been going well. Being able to stop, and take a few deep breaths will release the tensions of the body and will help you to get things back into perspective.

In my classes I suggest various images to help my students learn to relax. Use the ones you like and add others that occur to you as you relax. The feeling you are after is one of awareness without conscious thought, peacefulness, and a muscular release of all tensions in the body. You can relax in any position that's comfortable. You can sit in a semireclining position on your couch, chair, or bed with a pillow or two under your head and shoulders and another under your knees to relax your lower back. Lying on your side is also fine.

Begin by simply breathing deeply and restfully. Feel your abdomen and rib cage expand as they fill with air, and then gently allow the air to sail out through your lips as you exhale. Feel your body soften as you relax.

As you breathe, feel the gentle rise and fall of the body like the ebb and flow of the tide at the ocean.

Allow the floor to support you and let it absorb the weight of your body.

Feel your body soften and melt into the floor like an ice-cream cone on a warm day or butter in a saucepan on a warm stove.

Let a feeling of warmth and heaviness travel upward through your body as you let your toes hang from your feet, your feet hang from your ankles, your calves hang loosely from your knees, and your thighs hang open and soft from your hips.

Feel your forehead become smooth and calm. Also smooth the space between the eyes and eyebrows. Let your eyes rest.

Feel as though your body is a bag of sand, and feel the sand sift out of the body and into the floor. Imagine loose seams at the shoulders, the sides of the body, the palms and the soles of the feet, and the back of the neck. Let the bag empty.

Let your jaw soften and let your lips and teeth part slightly.

Let sounds enter and drift through your consciousness.

Recall a recent event or sensation that made you happy. Feel a smile come to your lips, then feel the smile spread to your entire face. Now let that smile permeate your whole body and smile with your whole body.

Become aware of the air underneath you, above you, and around you. Feel that you can breathe directly into and out of all the pores of the skin, and feel the air travel through you. Become light and one with the air.

Let thoughts enter and drift through your mind. Don't follow your thoughts. Instead, watch them go.

Allow a feeling of deep calm and contentment to permeate your mind and body.

Before getting up or proceeding to any exercises, take a minute or two to slowly stretch all the limbs of the body, reaching your legs long and away from you, and stretching your arms above your head. Stretch first one side of the body and then the other. Yawns feel good and are a natural response to stretching. Allow it to happen.

If you have the time, add a special period of relaxation as part of your daily exercise program. If not, include it only on those days you feel particularly tense in place of some of the exercises. Try some of the images at work when you can't get a nap or at night when you have trouble falling asleep.

When you exercise, think about incorporating the principles of relaxation. When a part of your body isn't moving and isn't needed to work, try consciously to relax it. Again, use the images to help you. For example, when your body is bent over your leg in the Leg Stretch With Twist (page 40), think about keeping your shoulders, neck, spine, and jaw relaxed as you flex and point your foot. When you do the Sitting Side Stretches (page 60), let your head drop to the side and relax the bottom shoulder as you stretch the opposite arm and side. The best way to move is the most efficient way to move—if you don't need it, don't use it!

V THE PRENATAL EXERCISES

The Prenatal Routines

Routine I

1. Pelvic Tilt
2. Side Knee Drops
3. Leg Stretches
4. Back Massage
5. Side Leg Lifting
6. Head Circles
7. Leg Stretch With Twist
8. Thigh Stretch

Routine II

1. Single Leg Slide
2. Side Press
3. Body Circles
4. Footwork
5. Hamstring Stretch
6. Open Pelvic Tilt
7. Side Leg Stretches
8. Side Stretch in Stride

Routine III

1. Sitting Side Stretches
2. Ankle Circles
3. Sitting Pelvic Tilt
4. Leg Stretches Opening Side
5. V-Stretch
6. Arm Circles
7. Body Twist
8. Graham Stretch

Prenatal Standing Exercise I
Prenatal Standing Exercise II
Prenatal Standing Exercise III
A Longer Prenatal Routine

| PRENATAL
ROUTINE

1. Pelvic Tilt

PURPOSE: To strengthen the abdominal and pelvic floor muscles
and to lengthen and relax the lower back.

TO START: Lie on the floor with your knees bent and the soles of
your feet on the floor, about hip width apart. Place
your hands either on your abdomen or straight down
by your sides.

INHALE deeply.

EXHALE: Contract your abdominal muscles so your belly tight-
ens and flattens, and feel your spine lengthen to the
floor. Now also tighten your pelvic floor muscles, but
keep your buttocks relaxed.

INHALE: Relax your pelvis completely. Feel your abdomen expand as it fills with air.

TOTAL: Six times.

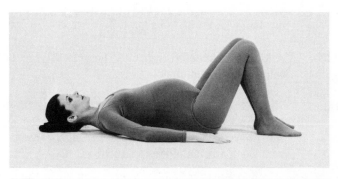

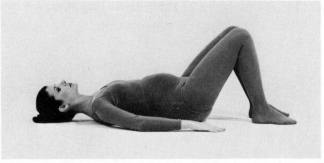

| PRENATAL
| ROUTINE

2. Side Knee Drops

PURPOSE: To relax the hips and lower back, and to tone the waist and abdominals.

NOTE: Try to do this exercise in one smooth, continuous motion, inhaling and exhaling, dropping the knees first to one side, and then the other, and massaging your lower back against the floor as you pass through center.

TO START: Lie on the floor with your knees bent and the soles of your feet on the floor, about hip width apart. Place your arms straight out to your sides, just below shoulder height.

INHALE: Allow your knees to relax to the side so your bottom thigh touches the floor.

EXHALE: Using the abdominal muscles, do a pelvic tilt to get your hips back to center. Feel your back flat against the floor each time you pass through center. Keep your neck and shoulders relaxed.

TOTAL: Six times to each side, alternating sides each time.

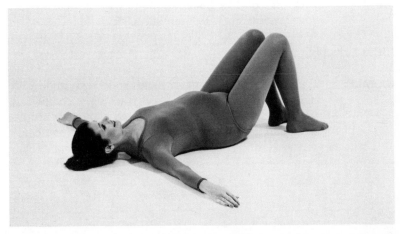

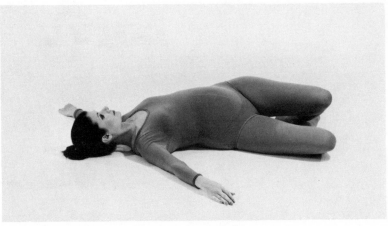

**❙ PRENATAL
❙ ROUTINE**

3. Leg Stretches I

PURPOSE: To tone and strengthen the muscles in the legs, feet, and abdomen.

TO START: Lie on the floor with your knees bent and the soles of your feet on the floor, about hip width apart. Rest your arms straight by your sides.

INHALE deeply.

EXHALE: Tighten your abdominal muscles and slowly slide your right foot along the floor until your leg is completely straight. Make sure your neck and shoulders are relaxed and that your lower back stays flat on the floor.

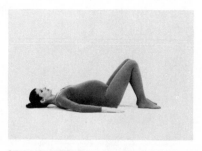

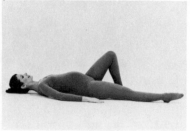

INHALE: Lift your leg off the floor, toward the ceiling. Try to use the muscles along the back of your leg, which is where you should feel the stretch. Only lift your leg to a comfortable height so that your buttocks stay on the floor.

EXHALE: Flex your foot, tighten your abdominal muscles, and slowly lower your heel to the floor. Keep lengthening your leg and heel away from your body—you'll get a better stretch and your leg won't feel so heavy.

INHALE: Relax your leg back to the starting (bent-knee) position.

TOTAL: Five times on each leg, alternating sides each time.

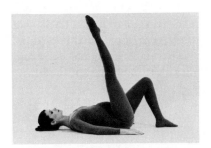

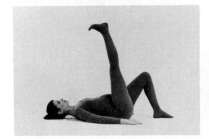
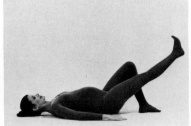

| PRENATAL
| ROUTINE

4. Back Massage

PURPOSE: To strengthen the abdominal muscles and to relax, lengthen, and increase flexibility in the spine. (This exercise is especially good for relieving lower back ache.)

TO START: Lie on the floor with your knees bent and the soles of your feet on the floor, about hip width apart. Place your arms straight down by your sides.

INHALE deeply.

EXHALE: Do a pelvic tilt then slowly peel your back off the floor, one vertebra at a time, lifting your lower back, then your waist, middle back, and finally your upper spine. Use your abdominals, your back, and the backs of your thighs to lift you up, and keep your lower back long and relaxed. *Do not arch your back.* If this is done correctly, there will be a straight, diagonal line from your shoulders to your knees at the height of the lift.

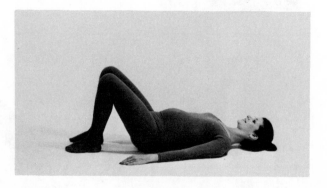

INHALE deeply.

EXHALE: Slowly roll your spine, one vertebra at a time, back to
           the floor, as if you had one strip of Velcro along your
           spine and another on the floor, and you wanted to
           match them evenly.

TOTAL: Six times.

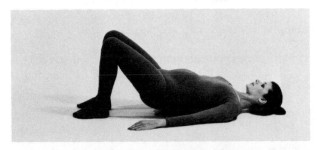

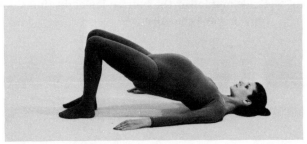

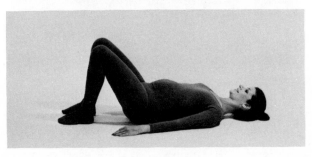

5. Side Leg Lifting

PURPOSE: To tone the waist, hips, and legs.

TO START: Lie on your side with your body on one straight line. Toes can either be pointed, or flexed, whichever you prefer. Lift the top leg to hip height.

INHALE deeply.

EXHALE: Tighten your abdominals to help you and lift the bottom leg to touch the top one. Think of bringing the inner thighs together, not the feet.

INHALE: Lower the bottom leg only.

TOTAL: Raise and lower the bottom leg eight times, lower the top leg, then change sides.

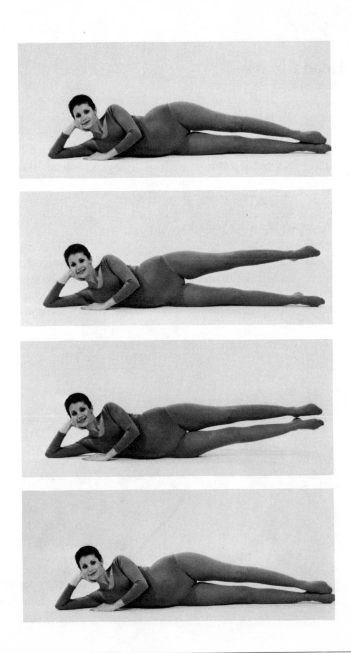

| PRENATAL
| ROUTINE

6. Head Circles

PURPOSE: To relax and stretch the upper back, neck, and shoulders.

TO START: Sit tailor fashion with your legs crossed. Rest your hands on your knees. Relax your neck and let your chin drop toward your chest.

BREATHE slowly and naturally throughout.

Slowly roll your head in circles, first in one direction and then the other. Relax your neck completely as you circle your head and feel the weight of your head stretch all the muscles around your neck and shoulders.

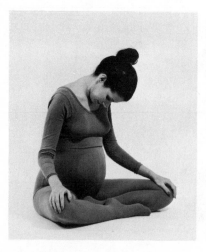 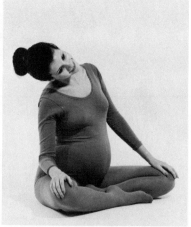

The shoulders have a tendency to lift during this exercise, so try consciously to keep them still by using opposition. As your head circles to the right, pull your left shoulder down; let both shoulders relax as your head drops back; pull your right shoulder down as your head circles to the left side. (This coordination of the head and shoulder will create a much stronger and deeper stretch.)

TOTAL: Four circles in each direction.

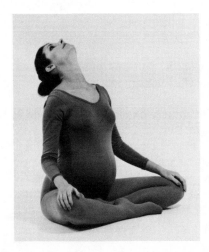 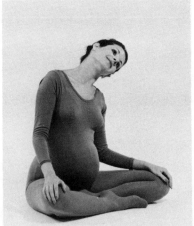

| PRENATAL
| ROUTINE

7. Leg Stretch With Twist

PURPOSE: To stretch and tone the entire body.

NOTE: This is a more difficult exercise, requiring many different positions, but it'll make you feel great!

TO START: Sit with your right leg straight out in front of you with your left knee bent and your left foot placed against the inside of your right thigh. Rest your right hand on your right leg and reach your left arm behind you.

INHALE: Stretch your left arm to the ceiling.

EXHALE: Round your spine and relax your left arm to the floor by your right leg as you relax your body over your right thigh. Let your shoulders and elbows soften. Relax your neck and jaw. (If you have trouble breathing while bent over, try keeping your back straight and lengthening your ribs away from your hips as you stretch forward. You'll still get the same stretch through the back of your leg.)

INHALE: Keep your body relaxed as you flex your right foot. Feel the stretch along the back of your right leg.

EXHALE: Point your right foot and relax your body lower to your leg.

INHALE: Reach your left arm to your right toes and stretch your spine longer as you open your body to face the side wall. Let your left arm follow naturally until it is extended next to your left ear. Your right side should be next to your right leg.

EXHALE: Tighten your abdominal muscles and roll your spine back to center. Feel both "sit bones" evenly on the floor underneath you. Allow your left arm to reach to the ceiling and back behind you, and your right arm to slide back to your right knee, returning both arms to the starting position.

TOTAL: Four times on each side.

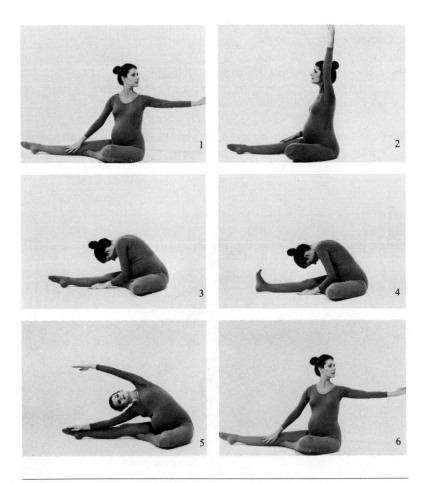

8. Thigh Stretch

PURPOSE: To stretch and lengthen the muscles in the front of the hips and thighs.

NOTE: If, while doing this exercise, you feel pain in your knees or if you have a history of knee problems, omit this movement from your routine.

TO START: Sit on your heels and place your arms comfortably behind you for support, palms flat on the floor.

INHALE deeply.

EXHALE: Tighten your abdominal and buttock muscles and gently lift your hips off your heels. Your back should be long and straight, not arched.

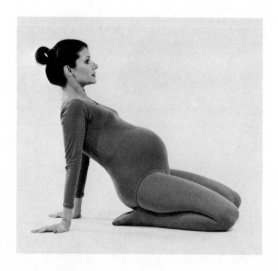

INHALE: Gently lower your hips back to your feet.

TOTAL: Six times.

END: Open your knees wide apart and relax all the way forward. You'll have to experiment to find the best position for your arms and body. You may want to rest your forehead or cheek on your hands (as shown) or to rest your forehead directly on the floor and relax your arms by your legs. Remain in this position for a minute or so, breathing slowly and deeply, and relaxing your back. Then slowly unroll your spine to straight, so that you're once again sitting on your heels.

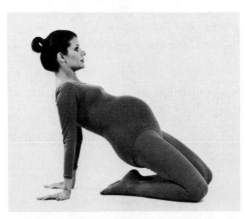

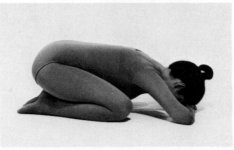

II PRENATAL ROUTINE

1. Single Leg Slide

PURPOSE: To tone and strengthen the muscles in the legs and abdomen.

TO START: Lie on the floor with your knees bent and the soles of your feet on the floor, about hip width apart. Rest your arms by your sides.

INHALE deeply.

EXHALE: Tighten your abdominal muscles and slowly slide your right foot along the floor until your leg is straight, using the buttocks and underneath muscles in your thigh. Feel very long and stretched from your head to your toes.

INHALE: Relax through your hip, knee, and ankle joints as you bend your knee back to the starting position.

TOTAL: Six times on each side, alternating legs each time.

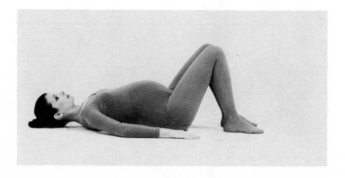

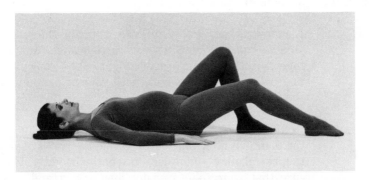

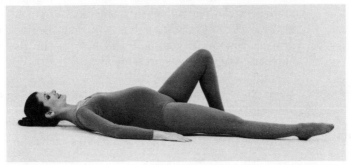

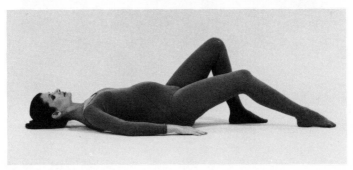

|| PRENATAL
|| ROUTINE

2. Side Press

PURPOSE: To tone the hips, waist, and thighs.

TO START: Lie on your back with your knees bent and the soles of
your feet on the floor. Start with your knees and feet
together. Place your arms straight out to your sides,
just below shoulder height, with your palms down to
the floor.

INHALE: Roll your hips to the right, touching your right knee to
the floor. Tighten your buttocks and the backs of your
thighs and allow your knees to separate slightly. Make
sure that your spine remains long and straight, not
arched, and that you push from the hips, not your
lower back. Feel the stretch across your shoulder and
arm as you press your left shoulder to the floor in
opposition to your hips pressing away.

EXHALE: Relax your hips and use the abdominal muscles to roll
your spine back to center.

TOTAL: Six times to each side, alternating sides each time.

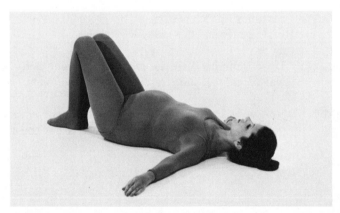

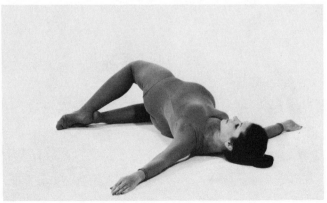

|| PRENATAL
|| ROUTINE

3. Body Circles

PURPOSE: To relax the neck, shoulder, and back and to tone the ribs and waistline.

NOTE: Each circle should be done in one continuous motion so that you move smoothly through (rather than stopping at) each position as shown.

TO START: Sit tailor fashion with your legs crossed. Let your hands rest lightly on your knees.

INHALE: Drop your head to the right, bend your body at the waist, and feel the stretch along your left side.

EXHALE: Roll your body forward so your back is rounded and your chin is in toward your chest. Feel the stretch along your back.

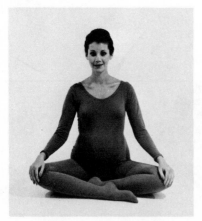 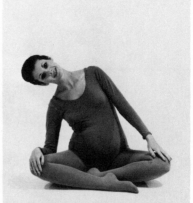

INHALE: Continue the circle to the left side, so your body is now leaning to the left and you feel the stretch along your right side.

EXHALE: Tighten your abdominals and roll up to the starting position.

TOTAL: Six circles to each direction.

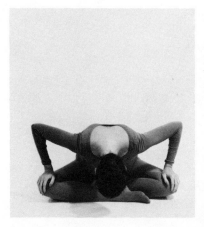 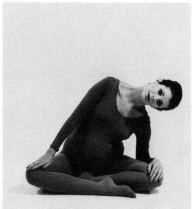

|| PRENATAL
|| ROUTINE

4. Footwork

PURPOSE: To improve the circulation and to stretch and tone the muscles in the legs and feet.

TO START: Sit with your legs straight in front of you and your arms slightly behind you for support, palms flat on floor, fingers extended straight back. Use the muscles in your back to maintain a straight spine.

BREATHE slowly and naturally throughout.

Flex your feet, bending your toes back toward you and straightening, stretching, and lengthening the backs of your legs, from your hips, through your knees, to your heels.

Then point your feet, stretching and lengthening the top muscles of your legs, from your thighs, through your knees, to the arches of your feet, and out through your toes. Lengthen your feet as you point.

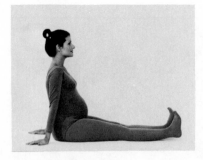 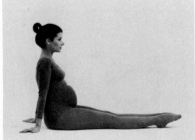

Also, try bending your knees as you flex your feet, and straightening them as you point your feet. In this way you can stretch your calves without involving the backs of the knees.

TOTAL: Eight times flexing, eight times pointing.

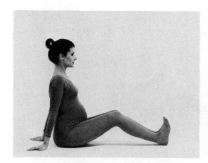 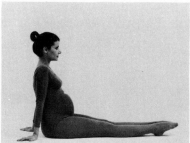

II PRENATAL ROUTINE

5. Hamstring Stretch

PURPOSE: To stretch the backs of the legs (called the hamstring
           muscles).

NOTE: Parts I and II should be done one right after the other
           before changing sides.

TO START: Lie on your back with your right leg straight and your
           left knee in toward your chest to the left side of your
           belly. Hold your left leg just below (not on) your knee.

Part I

INHALE: Feel your abdomen rise toward your thigh as it fills
           with air. Think of breathing into the lowest part of
           your pelvis, relaxing and softening the area around
           your left hip.

EXHALE: Tighten your abdominal muscles and allow your left
           leg to relax closer to your body.

BREATHE in this position for about a minute or two.

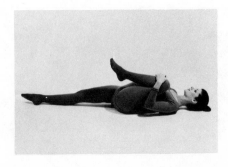

Part II

Now bend your right knee and straighten your left leg toward the ceiling.

INHALE: Flex your left foot and bend your left knee in to your chest.

EXHALE: *Try* to leave your thigh where it is (it's hard and your leg may tremble) and again, slowly, straighten your leg, keeping the foot flexed and pressing your heel toward the ceiling. Now point your foot. Let go of your leg if you need to.

TOTAL: Bend and straighten your leg four times, then repeat the entire exercise from Part I on the other side.

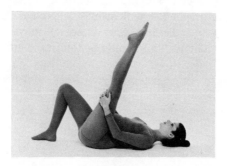

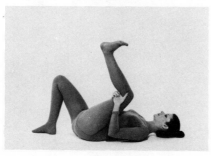

‖ PRENATAL
‖ ROUTINE

6. Open Pelvic Tilt

PURPOSE: To strengthen the abdominal, pelvic floor, and inner thigh muscles and to lengthen and relax the lower back.

TO START: Lie on the floor with your knees bent and dropped open to the sides and the soles of your feet together, as close to your body as possible. Place your arms straight down by your sides.

INHALE deeply.

EXHALE: Tighten your abdominal muscles so your belly flattens, and feel your spine lengthen and flatten to the floor. Tighten your pelvic floor muscles, too. *Press your heels together* and allow your knees to move toward each other a little. This should be felt in the inner thighs.

INHALE: Relax your hips and let your knees gently drop open.

TOTAL: Six times.

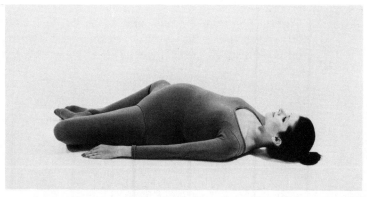

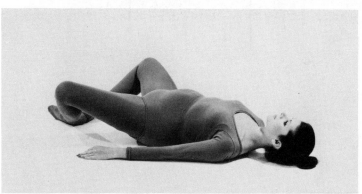

‖ PRENATAL
‖ ROUTINE

7. Side Leg Stretches

PURPOSE: To tone and firm the legs.

TO START: Lie on your left side in one straight line, left arm
              extended straight, palm down on floor. Rest your head
              on your left arm. Place your right hand palm down on
              the floor next to your chest for balance.

INHALE: Bend your right knee up toward the ceiling.

EXHALE: Tighten your abdominals and buttocks, and slowly
              straighten your right leg. Work to keep your leg turned
              out from your hip so that the inside of your thigh faces
              outward.

INHALE: Flex your right foot and stretch both legs longer.

EXHALE: Tighten your abdominals and buttocks and slowly lower
              your leg, lengthening and keeping it as turned out as
              much as possible as it lowers.

TOTAL: Eight times on each leg.

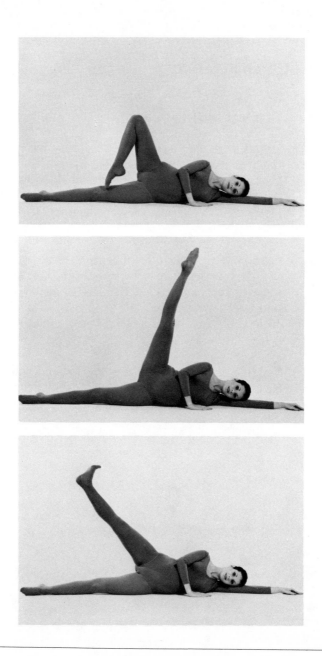

|| PRENATAL
|| ROUTINE

8. Side Stretch in Stride

PURPOSE: To stretch and tone the entire body.

TO START: Sit tall, with your legs straight and *comfortably* open.
            Don't worry if you don't look like the model—just *feel*
            like her. Reach your arms out to your sides, just below
            shoulder height. Stretch your legs and feet longer and
            rotate your thighs open, so your legs are "turned out"
            from your hips.

INHALE: Place your right hand on your right ankle or calf and
            stretch your left arm over your head, bending side-
            ways at your waist. Feel the stretch along your left
            side as you stretch your left hand and foot in opposite
            directions. Make sure both hips stay squarely on the
            floor.

EXHALE: Tighten your abdominal muscles and roll your body
            back to center. Feel both sit bones evenly underneath
            you.

TOTAL: Four times to each side, alternating sides each time.

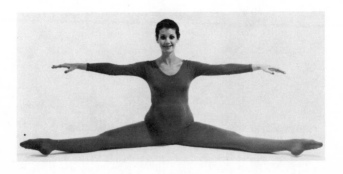

END: Place your hands on the floor in front of you and round your spine. Breathe slowly and deeply and let your body, head, neck, shoulders, arms, and legs relax. Allow your inner thighs to stretch gently. Stay in this position for about two minutes, then slowly round your spine up to sitting. Bring your legs together and shake them out by gently bouncing them up and down against the floor.

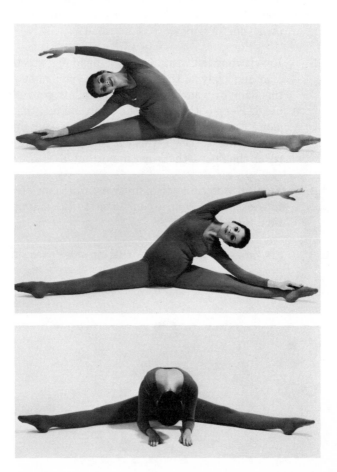

III PRENATAL ROUTINE

1. Sitting Side Stretches

PURPOSE: To tone and firm the arms, waist, ribs, and back.

TO START: Sit tailor fashion with your legs crossed and your arms out by your sides so your fingertips just touch the floor. Feel the weight of your body centered and even over your sit bones.

INHALE: Reach your left arm over your head and stretch your arm and body to the right. Place your right palm on the floor by your right side and allow your elbow to bend. Keep both hips on the floor and feel the stretch along the left side of your body, from your fingertips to your waist. (Don't worry if your right elbow doesn't reach the floor—that's not important.)

EXHALE: Tighten your abdominal muscles, roll your left side up to center, and return your arms to the starting position. Sit tall.

TOTAL: Six times to each side, alternating sides each time.

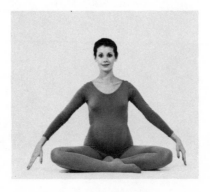

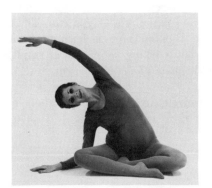

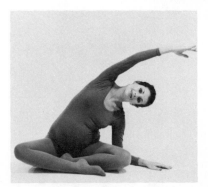

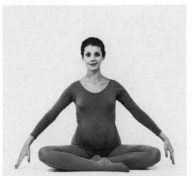

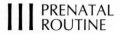

III PRENATAL ROUTINE

2. Ankle Circles

PURPOSE: To improve the circulation and to stretch and tone the muscles in the legs and feet.

TO START: Either lie flat on your back, or lean back on your elbows (as shown), with both knees bent. Take your right leg and place the calf across your left knee.

BREATHE slowly and naturally throughout.

Slowly circle your foot, flexing and pointing, and making as full a circle as you can. Try to move only your foot, working the muscles in your foot, ankle, and calf, but not working your knee or thigh. By the end, your ankle should feel quite warm.

TOTAL: Ten circles in each direction, then change legs.

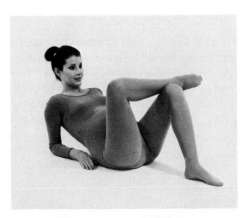

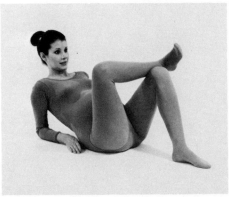

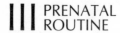 PRENATAL
ROUTINE

3. Sitting Pelvic Tilt

PURPOSE: To tone and strengthen the abdominal and pelvic floor muscles, and to stretch the inner thighs.

TO START: Sit with the soles of your feet together and close to your body, and your knees wide apart. Put your hands on your ankles.

INHALE deeply.

EXHALE: Strongly tighten and flatten your abdomen and allow your *lower* back to round. Try to keep your rib cage high so you don't slump as you work your abdominals. Tighten your pelvic floor muscles at the same time.

INHALE: Gently relax your abdominal and pelvic floor muscles and grow taller as you use your back to lift your body back to center. You may use your hands on your ankles to help you, also.

TOTAL: Six times.

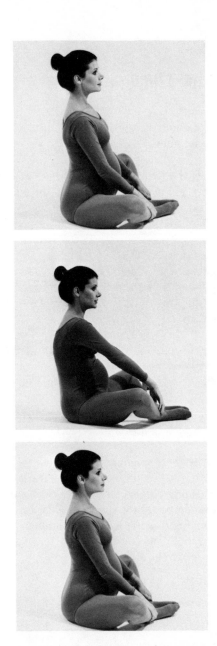

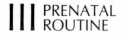 PRENATAL
ROUTINE

4. Leg Stretches Opening Side

PURPOSE: To tone and strengthen the muscles in the legs, feet, and abdomen.

TO START: Lie on the floor with your knees bent and the soles of your feet on the floor, about hip width apart. Rest your arms straight down by your sides.

INHALE deeply.

EXHALE: Tighten your abdominal muscles and slowly slide your right foot along the floor until your leg is completely straight, toes pointed. Keep your lower back flat to the floor.

INHALE: Stretch your leg off the floor toward the ceiling and feel the stretch along the back of your leg. *Keep your buttocks on the floor* and lift your leg to a comfortable height, keeping your right knee straight. Don't worry if your leg doesn't go as high as pictured—stretch comes with time and practice.)

EXHALE: Tighten your abdominals, flex your right foot, and open your leg to the side. Rotate the inside of your thigh to the ceiling. Make sure both hips stay on the floor. What's important is the outward rotation of the moving leg and the work in the abdominals in keeping your lower back on the floor, not how low you can take your leg to the side.

INHALE: Point your foot and stretch your leg toward the ceiling.

EXHALE: Tighten your abdominals and lower your leg to the floor.

INHALE: Bend your knee back to the starting position.

TOTAL: Four times on each side, alternating legs each time.

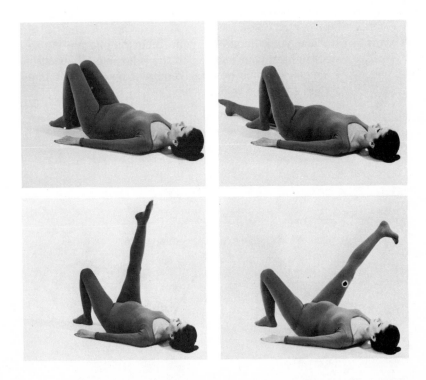

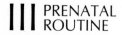 PRENATAL
ROUTINE

5. V-Stretch

PURPOSE: To tone and strengthen the abdomen, legs, and feet.

TO START: Lie on your back with your knees bent in toward your chest. Place your hands on your legs just below your knees.

INHALE: Open your knees wide, place your feet together, and slide your hands down the insides of your legs to your ankles. Use your hands to pull your feet closer to you, and use your elbows against your knees to press them wider apart.

EXHALE: Place your hands on your inner thighs and *slowly* straighten your legs out to the sides in a "V" position. The legs should be rotated outward, so that the inner thighs face the ceiling.

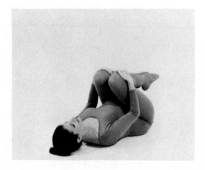 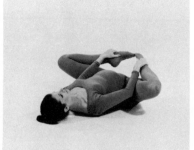

INHALE: Using the inner thighs, bring your legs together.

EXHALE: Gently bend your knees back in toward your chest.

TOTAL: Six times.

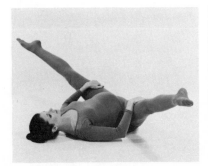 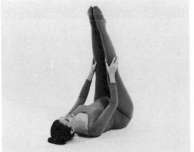

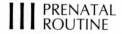 **PRENATAL ROUTINE**

6. Arm Circles

PURPOSE: To tone and strengthen the muscles in the back, arms, and chest.

NOTE: Your arms should move slowly and with resistance through this exercise, as if they were underwater. Feel your arms working from the muscles in your back and sides, not from your shoulders.

TO START: Sit tailor fashion with your legs crossed. Place your arms by your sides.

INHALE: Reach your arms forward, elbows straight.

EXHALE: Press your shoulders down and lift your arms above your head.

INHALE: Circle your arms behind you and press your shoulder blades together in the back.

EXHALE: Return your arms back to the starting position.

TOTAL: Eight circles in each direction.

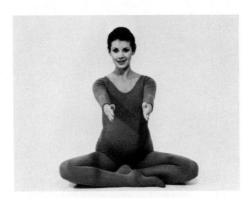

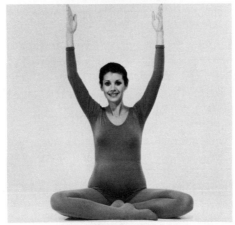

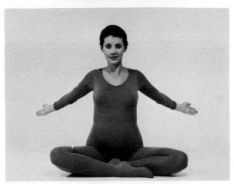

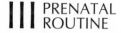 PRENATAL
ROUTINE

7. Body Twist

PURPOSE: To stretch and tone the waist and upper body and to increase flexibility in the back.

NOTE: This exercise can be done slowly, maintaining the twist and breathing as you stay in the one position, or more quickly, changing sides with each breath. Try doing it both ways and see which you prefer.

TO START: Sit tailor fashion with your legs crossed.

INHALE: Place your right hand on your left knee and your left palm on the floor next to your spine. Keep your left elbow straight.

EXHALE: Twist your ribs to the left, using your right hand to help you. Look over your left shoulder.

INHALE: Change hands and twist to the right. Your left hand should now be on your right knee and you should be looking over your right shoulder.

TOTAL: Six times to each direction.

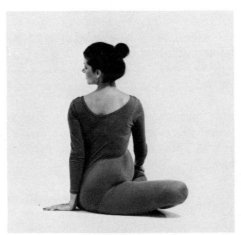

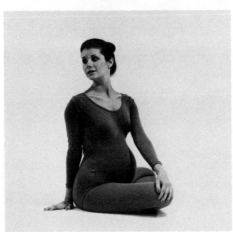

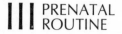 PRENATAL
ROUTINE

8. Graham Stretch
(Adapted from a Martha Graham dance warm-up)

PURPOSE: To tone and stretch the entire body, especially the muscles in the legs and back.

TO START: Sit in a comfortable stride position so that your legs are wide apart. Place your hands either on your thighs or on the floor in front of you.

INHALE deeply.

EXHALE: Pull your abdomen in and allow your lower back to round in response. Flex your feet and rotate your thighs open in the hip sockets. Keep your knees straight.

INHALE: Round your back and relax your body toward the floor. Keep your feet flexed and rotated open. Feel the stretch in your back and inner thighs.

EXHALE: Point your toes. Maintaining this forward position, slowly straighten your spine, starting at the lowest vertebra and working your way up, in sequence, to the top of your neck until your body is on one straight diagonal line. You may need to check yourself in a mirror. Make sure your shoulders are down and that your neck is in line with the rest of your spine.

INHALE: Lift your body back to center.

TOTAL: Six times.

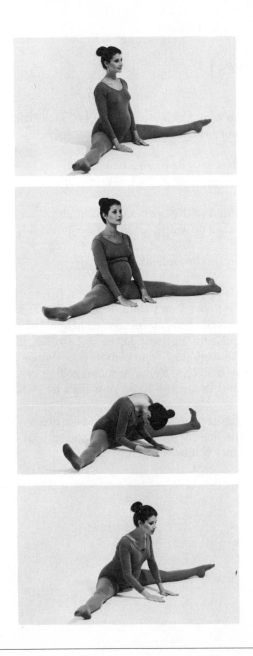

PRENATAL STANDING EXERCISE

Pliés/Relevés I

PURPOSE: To tone the entire body, but especially the legs and inner thighs.

NOTE: Dancers often use a ballet barre, so feel free to hold on to a chair or wall while doing this exercise.

TO START: Stand with your feet comfortably apart and your toes facing outward, arms down comfortably at your sides.

BREATHE naturally throughout.

TO PLIÉ: Slowly bend your knees open, *but keep your heels on the floor.* Don't think of going down, however. Think instead of maintaining your height and simply reaching and bending your knees out to the sides. Make sure the weight of your body is distributed evenly through both feet, so that you're not rolling inward or outward on your arches. Keep your back long and straight.

Tighten your abdominals and press your heels into the floor as you slowly straighten your legs. Feel your inner thighs working.

TO RELEVÉ: Press your toes and the balls of your feet into the floor and press your heels off the floor. Use your inner thighs and abdominals to help your body balance over your feet. Try to keep that tall as you slowly (and with control from the inner thighs and abdominals) lower your heels to the floor.

TOTAL: Six times, alternating pliés with relevés.

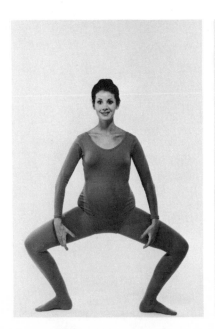
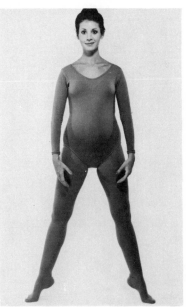

‖ PRENATAL
‖ STANDING EXERCISE

Table Top I

PURPOSE: To stretch and tone the entire body.

TO START: Stand with your feet comfortably apart.

INHALE: Stretch your arms above your head, keeping your shoulders down.

EXHALE: (Keeping your back straight, stretch your body forward from the hips like a Barbie plastic doll) until your back is parallel to the floor (or as close to parallel as your individual flexibility allows). Keep your neck and arms in line with your spine, and check yourself in a mirror if you can.

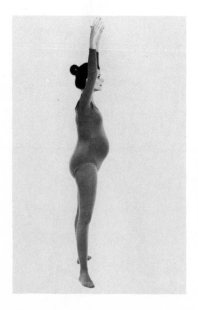 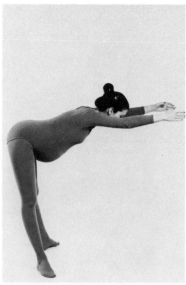

INHALE: Let your back round and relax your body toward the floor. Keep your knees straight, and feel the stretch along the backs of your legs. It is *not* important to be able to touch the floor.

EXHALE: Tighten your abdomen and slowly unroll your spine, vertebra by vertebra, to standing.

TOTAL: Four times.

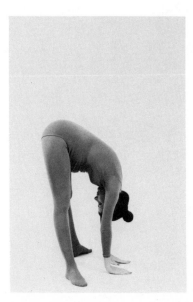 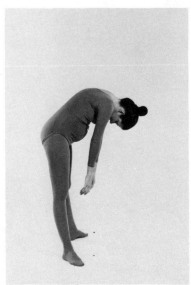

III PRENATAL STANDING EXERCISE

Standing Side Stretch I

PURPOSE: To stretch and tone the entire body.

TO START: Stand with your legs comfortably apart and your toes facing outward. Reach your arms straight out to your sides just below shoulder height, palms down.

INHALE: Bend your left knee, let your head drop to the left, and bend your body sideways at the waist. Stretch your right arm over your head and reach with both arms out to the left.

EXHALE: Tighten your abdomen, straighten your left knee, and lift your body back to center.

TOTAL: Four times to each side, alternating sides each time.

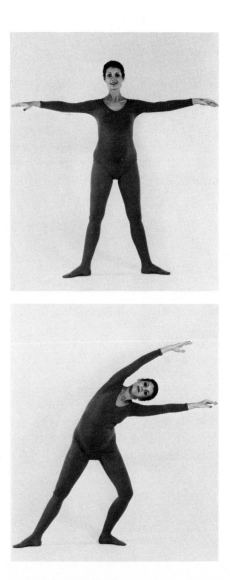

A LONGER PRENATAL EXERCISE ROUTINE

If you would like to exercise for an hour instead of the fifteen or twenty minutes each of the suggested routines takes, try doing all of the prenatal exercises, in the following order. They are arranged so that you will begin with the simpler and easier movements and progress to those that are more strenuous, warming your muscles gradually.

They are also arranged so that different parts of your body will be worked on successive exercises, alternating exercises for the legs, arms, feet, and upper body. You will also be alternating sitting exercises with the ones when you are on your back side so that muscles are not fatigued by being in one position for any great length of time.

1. Pelvic Tilt (pg. 28)
2. Single Leg Slide (pg. 44)
3. Leg Stretches I (pg. 32)
4. Side Knee Drops (pg. 30)
5. Leg Stretches Opening Side (pg. 66)
6. Open Pelvic Tilt (pg. 54)
7. Side Leg Lifting (pg. 36)
8. Body Circles (pg. 48)
9. Footwork (pg. 50)
10. Sitting Pelvic Tilt (pg. 64)
11. Body Twist (pg. 72)
12. Ankle Circles (pg. 62)
13. Side Stretch in Stride (pg. 58)
14. V-Stretch (pg. 68)

VI COMMON PREGANCY PROBLEMS AND CONCERNS

Pregnancy is a time of myriad physical changes. The breasts enlarge, the body grows rounder, and the abdomen expands, making room for the baby as it grows. The uterus presses against the stomach and ribs causing heartburn and shortness of breath. It displaces the intestines and other internal organs making digestion more difficult, constipation a problem, and creating a need to urinate more frequently. These changes can also cause concern. One wants to know if certain aches and pains are "normal" and if anyone else has them, too. My students come to my classes for exercise, but just being with and talking to other pregnant women is an important part, also. In fact, there are times I think they'd rather stay in the dressing room and talk than begin class! It's a relief to share concerns with other pregnant women and to discover that they have experienced the same sensations.

The following is a brief discussion of some of these concerns, and answers to the most frequently asked questions regarding common pregnancy complaints.

WEIGHT GAIN AND ABDOMINAL SIZE

I'm including a few words about weight gain and abdominal size because I see such a great deal of anxiety among my students on the subject. They ask each other what month they're in and how much weight they've gained so far. They compare belly sizes and exchange comments about how "large" or "small" their bellies seem. One student will jokingly ask a newcomer to the class who's barely "showing" if she's sure she's really pregnant. (Although meant as a compliment, this can also be upsetting to the new student.) Most women are concerned about their changing figures and their weight gain. They worry that if they gain seven or eight pounds in one month they will continue to gain at that rate for the rest of the pregnancy. They wonder how much of what they are gaining is baby and how much is fat, and about being able to lose any extra weight after the baby is born. Other women are concerned when people remark on how "small" they look, and worry if the baby is growing adequately.

Unfortunately, women get a great deal of conflicting advice from many different sources. One friend may warn that she'd better be careful because it's hard to lose the weight afterward (which it isn't), while another will warn her that her appetite is a sign from her baby and body that they need food and that she should eat as much as she wants. Even physicians are not always in agreement. Some doctors believe in restricting the weight gain while others allow much more leeway. It can be very confusing trying to figure out what's "right."

There is no absolute "right" or "wrong," only what's right or wrong for you. Every woman and every baby will gain weight at different rates during the nine months of pregnancy. You may gain a steady two to four pounds each month, but more likely you will gain more weight some months than others. Many women experience a larger weight gain, as much as eight to ten pounds, around the fourth or fifth month and much smaller weight gains at the very beginning and at the very end of the pregnancy. The *average* weight gain by the end of the ninth month is anywhere from twenty-five to thirty pounds, but there are many women who gain more or less depending on a wide range of factors such as the weight and size of the baby(s), the amount of amniotic fluid, and the size of the placenta. Women who are very slim at the onset of pregnancy seem to need to gain more weight, while others who were slightly overweight may gain less.

Try not to be overly concerned with the amount of weight you gain, and use your common sense. If you're in your fifth month and you've already gained thirty pounds or you've only gained five, there may be reason to be concerned. But if your weight gain has *averaged* around two to four pounds per month, you're probably doing fine.

The size of your abdomen will also depend on many of these same factors. It makes sense that women with larger babies will probably also have larger bellies. The amount of amniotic fluid and the size of the placenta will also affect the size of your abdomen. One woman I know was quite large by the end of her pregnancy and everyone was convinced she was going to have a big baby. As it turned out, her baby weighed a very average seven pounds eleven ounces, but she had a huge placenta.

A woman's height and the length of her torso also affect the size of her abdomen. Women who are tall tend to "show" later and to "carry smaller" because they simply have more internal "room" for the baby. On the other hand, if the woman is tall, but so is her husband, she may be carrying a ten-pound baby by the end of her pregnancy and be just as large as her five foot two neighbor.

Understand that concern about the size of your abdomen and the amount of weight you're gaining may be a reflection of anxiety about your changing body. Many women go through a period in their pregnancies when they feel more "fat" than pregnant. It's about this time that your regular clothes no longer fit but you're not yet ready for maternity outfits, either. The reality of the pregnancy may not be established and the most natural response to this growing body may be "gee, look how fat I'm getting!"

This phase can also be upsetting as your pregnancy seems to take over your body, changing it weekly. Most of us who are pregnant for the first time have never seen a pregnant body before and may be ambivalent in our feelings toward it. Is it pretty, strange, shapely, beautiful or a little of everything? Questions about whether you're still attractive to your mate are normal, as you both adjust to your new pregnant body.

This period soon passes, however, as you feel the baby move and as you begin to look, not just feel, pregnant. Soon pride and excitement will replace any early anxieties as you enjoy this new life within you and you look forward to meeting the new addition to your family.

Exercise will help you to feel good during this early period and throughout your pregnancy by keeping you in touch with your changing body and by helping you to maintain a positive self-image. Good posture habits and regular exercise will make you feel strong and energetic and you may never go through the phase described above. Instead, you will probably maintain that lovely pregnancy glow as you carry yourself and your baby with grace and ease.

Exercise will make you feel better and so will eating all those healthy and nutritious foods such as milk, fresh vegetables, fruit, and whole-grain breads.

It was once thought that the baby could extract from the mother's body what it needed no matter what the mother ate. It was also once thought that the placenta acted as a barrier to any harmful foods or medications the mother ingested. We now know that this is not the case and that the baby grows on nutrients the mother eats, not what she has stored in her body. We also know that everything the mother consumes (except a very few chemicals with large molecular structures) passes through the placenta to the baby.

So watch what you eat. Depending on the quantities consumed and the time during the pregnancy they are taken, cigarettes, coffee, drugs, and liquor can all be harmful to the baby. Eat eggs, cheese, salads, and fruit instead of candy, cookies, cake, and other high-calorie low-nutrition foods. You'll both be stronger and healthier for it.

You should really be more concerned about your diet than your weight gain since what you eat is far more important than how much you eat. If you like to nibble in the evenings while you read or watch television, do you snack on potato chips and cookies or apples and carrots? If you've gained three pounds this week and you've been eating meat, fish, vegetables, and fruit, it's very different than if you've been consuming a pint of ice cream and a box of cookies every night. In the first instance, the gain is probably due to the baby's gaining weight; in the second, the gain will probably show up on your waist and thighs.

It is essential that you know that both you and your baby are directly affected by what you eat. Pregnancy is *not* the time to lose weight. It's a great time, however, to watch what you eat and to make sure you eat correctly.

COMMON PREGNANCY COMPLAINTS

Below are some of the *most common problems*. Mostly, aches and pains come and go as one ache disappears and another one appears someplace else. I do feel strongly, however, that if you are really concerned about something, ask your doctor or midwife. Don't be timid about asking them questions—that's part of their job. Call, don't wait for your next prenatal visit. If there is something wrong, it's best to catch it early, and if it's one of those "normal" pregnancy complaints, you'll be reassured and have saved yourself days or even weeks of worry.

Leg Cramps

There are different theories as to why women get leg cramps during pregnancy. Some think it has to do with a deficiency in calcium or a disturbance in calcium metabolism, while others think it has to do with the slowing of blood circulation in the legs. If cramping is a problem, try increasing your intake of milk products (good sources of calcium) by eating more yogurt and cheese and drinking more milk. Also exercise your legs by doing Leg Stretches and Ankle Circles and Footwork. Keeping the muscles in your legs toned and supple should either eliminate the cramping completely or at least cut down on the frequency and strength of the cramps.

If you tend to get leg cramps, try to exercise your legs and feet not only during your daily routine, but whenever you can think of it—while you're on the telephone or watching TV, sitting on a bus or riding in a car.

When you get a leg cramp, don't massage it. Just relax the leg completely until it passes. Then put your leg under the bathtub

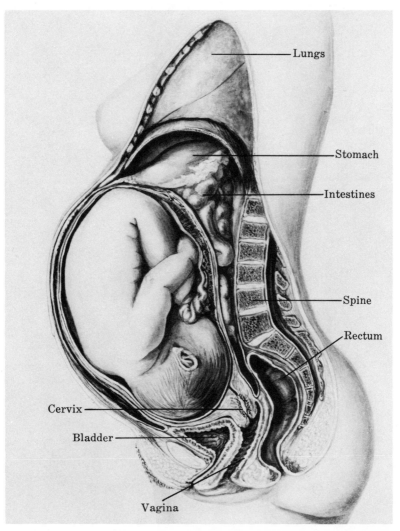

Courtesy of the Maternity Center Association

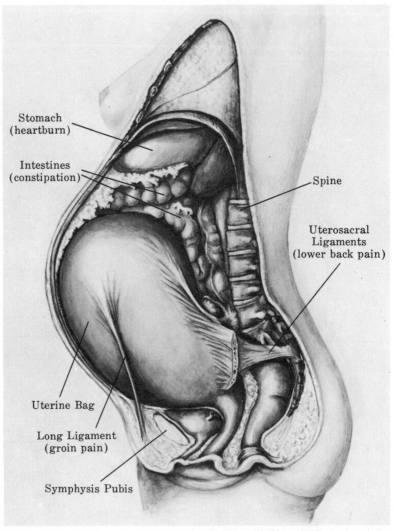

Courtesy of the Maternity Center Association

faucet (or use a hand shower-massage attachment) and run alternately hot then cold water directly on the muscles that cramped. This will stimulate circulation to the area and will ease the soreness that occurs afterward. Once the leg feels better, do slow stretches, flexing and pointing the foot. Any soreness from the cramp should pass within a day or two.

Varicose Veins

Varicose veins are veins which have become swollen due to an increase in pressure in the surrounding tissues. There is an inherited tendency toward varicose veins, but pregnancy is often the time when they first become pronounced.

Unfortunately, there is nothing that can be done to prevent them, although there are things you can do so they don't get worse. Elevate your legs as much and as often as possible, avoid standing in one place for any length of time, wear support hose, and exercise your legs by doing Leg Stretches I, Footwork, Ankle Circles, Leg Stretches Opening Side, and Side Leg Stretches.

Constipation

There are two very good reasons why constipation can be a problem during pregnancy. One, there is less room for the intestines as the uterus grows and there is more pressure on the bowel. Two, the hormones in the body which allow the stretching of the abdomen to occur also relax the smooth muscles of the bowels, so they work less efficiently.

For relief, drink lots of fluids (six to eight glasses of liquid each day—prune or other fruit juice, milk, water, etc.), eat whole-grain breads, add roughage (such as greens and celery) and include dried and fresh fruits in your diet (such as apples, prunes, dates, apricots, etc.). Exercise also helps.

Nausea

Nausea can be a problem at many times during one's pregnancy, but morning sickness usually disappears after the first trimester. For early morning nausea, keep dry crackers by your bedside and have a few when you first wake up. Wait a few minutes, then get out of bed slowly. Save your fruit juice (which is acidic) until *after* you have your breakfast.

The problem, however, is not always confined to the morning hours or to the first few months of pregnancy. Many women find they develop a sensitivity to certain odors such as perfumes, colognes, and cooking smells. If odors are a problem, try to keep to well-ventilated areas with fans, air-conditioning, or open windows. To relieve nausea, drink a cup of warm camomile or peppermint tea. If eating meals is a problem, don't try to finish an entire meal or a whole sandwich all at once. Nibble your food a little at a time, all day long. That way you'll still be getting the nutrition you need without having to force yourself to eat.

Heartburn

There are no miracle cures for heartburn (except giving birth), but you can try eating lots of small meals instead of two or three large ones, and bland foods rather than spicy or fried ones.

If it's a problem when you're trying to go to sleep at night, try putting a pillow or two under your head and shoulders so that you're not lying flat. You may find yourself sleeping in a semi-reclining position, but at least you'll be sleeping!

Antacids such as Mylanta, Rolaids, Maalox, and Milk of Magnesia, can also be taken if okayed by your doctor or midwife.

Sciatica

Sciatica is a very common problem during pregnancy and usually presents itself as pain (it can be either shooting or dull) in the buttocks, which can extend down the back of the thigh and leg to the ankle. It is caused by pressure from the uterus on the sciatic nerve. For some women this is a very temporary problem, relieved when the baby shifts to a different position, while for others, it is relieved only by the delivery of the baby.

Exercise, I'm sorry to admit, will not help sciatica. You cannot "work it out." You can continue doing any of the exercises that don't involve lifting the legs (such as Head Circles, Body Circles, Side Stretches, and Pelvic Tilts). You can also try doing the exercises "smaller"—that is, not lifting the leg as high as you usually do or not bending over as low.

Stop if it hurts. Your body is sending you a message that's plain and clear. If exercise is painful give it up. Take a hot bath instead, and try again another day. If you insist on exercising despite intense pain, you will only create more tension in your body and probably aggravate your condition.

Soreness or Sharp Pains in the Groin

During pregnancy the heavy uterine bag is supported by four different support systems: (1) the abdominal muscles, (2) the pelvic floor muscles, (3) the utero-sacral ligaments (which run from the uterus to the sacrum, or lower spine), and (4) the long ligaments.

The long ligaments run from the uterus to the pelvis and help support the uterus from underneath, like columns in a building. They hurt sometimes when you cough or sneeze because they are being suddenly stretched. You may even think you might have "pulled" something. Or they may start to hurt as you walk. Consciously tightening your abdominal muscles while you walk will not only give you better posture, but will also take some of the weight off those long ligaments and reduce that soreness in the groin. Tightening the belly when you sneeze or cough will also help.

Every once in a while I'll notice that a student of mine has suddenly begun to look very pregnant, and what used to be a little mound of belly has taken a more characteristically pregnant shape. This can even happen from one week to the next. I call it sprouting, because it reminds me of how a plant in the spring will grow one new leaf one day and by the end of the week be covered with new leaves. Growth spurts like these are common in pregnancy, but can cause some soreness (growing pains) as the supporting muscles and ligaments stretch.

There's not a great deal that can be done when soreness occurs except to take warm, leisurely baths. It helps, though, to know that it's only a temporary condition that will soon pass.

Lower Back Ache

Lower back ache can be a problem during pregnancy because of the extra work the muscles in the spine have to do to help support the weight of the fetus and uterine bag. Again, women with poor posture who let their bellies hang forward and who accentuate the curve in the lower back increase the strain. This can even be a problem in early pregnancy with women who push their bellies forward in the attempt to let others know they're pregnant.

To prevent lower back ache, refer to the instructions in the section on posture (page 19). Use your abdominal muscles to help support the uterus and try to remember to stand and walk tall at all times. Try *not* to look pregnant. Don't worry, you won't fool anybody, but you will benefit from improved posture and stronger abdominal muscles. Always let the back and buttocks relax and lift through the front of the body instead.

Exercise will also alleviate lower back ache, especially the Pelvic Tilt, Back Massage, Single Leg Slide, Side Knee Rolls, Body Circles, and Part I of the Hamstring Stretch.

VII CUT-OUT PAGES TO TAKE TO THE HOSPITAL

No matter what kind of delivery you have had, exercise will help you to feel better faster. The following exercises can be started hours after a vaginal birth or one day following a cesarean birth. They are gentle exercises and should be done every day during the first week following your delivery.

After the first week continue to do any of the prenatal exercises. Once you have your doctor or midwife's o.k., start the more strenuous postnatal program.

1. *Pelvic Floor Exercise*
Keep doing those pelvic floor exercises! It will help your episiotomy heal, if you've had one, and even if you haven't, it will help keep those perineal, vaginal, and rectal muscles toned and strong. Do them even if you've had a cesarean birth.

You may have trouble locating those muscles at first, but with a little practice, you'll be able to get them back to your prepregnancy tone (or better).

2. *Ankle Circles*
These are good to prevent swelling in your legs and to pro-

mote circulation. You can do them in your hospital bed with your legs out in front of you or with your legs hanging over the side.

Make lots of big circles with your feet, flexing and pointing them as they move. Circle your feet toward each other, then circle them away from each other, about eight times in each direction.

3. *Pelvic Tilt*

These will help to get your abdominals back in shape and will help to relax and stretch your lower back.

Lie on your bed with your knees bent and the soles of your feet on the mattress. Place your hands on your abdomen. Inhale deeply and feel your abdomen fill with air. Now exhale and tighten your abdominal muscles so you feel your abdomen flatten and your lower back press to the bed. Repeat seven more times.

4. *Single Leg Stretches*

These are also good for the circulation in your legs. Lie on your bed with both knees bent and the soles of your feet on the bed. Slowly straighten one leg at a time, inhaling as you bend your knee back to the starting position and exhaling as you slide the leg out. Start with four on each leg the first day, and add one more on each side each day after that.

5. *Head Circles*

Sit comfortably in a chair or on your bed. Breathe slowly and deeply as you gently roll your head around in a circle, first in one direction, and then in the other. This will feel very good, and will help to relax the muscles around your neck and shoulders.

VIII YOUR BODY AFTER BIRTH

I still remember the shock I felt on my first visit to a hospital maternity ward when I saw that new mothers still looked pregnant. Somehow I thought that once the baby was born, the abdomen just deflated like a balloon without air. But here I was confronted with all these women in bathrobes (whom I knew had delivered) all looking six months pregnant! I didn't know that it takes about six to eight weeks (or longer) for a woman to return to her prepregnancy body.

Most women are better informed than I was and expect a less drastic change following the birth of their babies. Many women, in fact, feel quite thin those first postpartum days in the hospital.

The average weight gain in pregnancy is about twenty-five to thirty pounds. Weight loss in the first two to ten days after birth is anywhere from ten to twenty pounds due to the expulsion of the baby and the placenta, to lower blood volume, and to fluid loss. The rest of the weight is distributed to the breasts and other parts of the body in preparation for breastfeeding.

Those first few days after birth include many physical changes as your body readjusts itself to its new, nonpregnant state. You'll probably have hot flashes or feel very warm. You may perspire a lot and need to change your nightgown and bed clothes quite often. You may also find you have to urinate frequently. This is normal, and is your body's natural way of excreting excess fluids that have accumulated during the pregnancy.

Your uterus will continue to contract in order to involute (or return to) its regular size (one-twentieth to one-twenty-fifth of its pregnancy size). These contractions are called "after pains" though they may not necessarily hurt, and you will probably be most aware of them as you breastfeed. Women who have had their second, third, or fourth child will probably feel these contractions more strongly than those who have had their first. Lying on your stomach with a pillow under your chest and shoulders will help your uterus to return to its home deep in the pelvis. (If you've had a cesarean birth, don't lie on your stomach until the stitches have been removed.)

Your episiotomy (if you've had one) may hurt. Put ice on it immediately after the birth to help prevent swelling. Then do *lots* of pelvic floor contractions to get the circulation going in the perineum and to promote healing. Most women find that after just a few days, the episiotomy is no longer uncomfortable. Others feel discomfort for up to a few months postpartum.

YOUR FIGURE

Once the uterus sinks into the pelvis, the postpartum body makes its appearance—heavy breasts, thick waist, and flabby belly. Remember, this is *very* temporary. Your body needs time to make its necessary adjustments. After all, you didn't get to be a nine months' size overnight, and you shouldn't expect your body to recover overnight either.

If you are tremendously overweight, you may want your doctor or nutritionist to work out a diet program for obvious health reasons. But if you simply have an extra five to ten pounds, I'd really encourage you to just let it be for a while. You have enough adjustments to make, just having an addition to the family—physically, mentally, and emotionally—without adding the additional burden of dieting. Exercise as often as you can starting with the day you deliver (see *cut-out page 95 for the hospital*) and give yourself at least six months before you attempt any serious dieting. Do not start a new exercise routine until you consult your doctor or midwife.

Breastfeeding will make a difference in how quickly you regain your figure. I have found that most women fall into one of two categories: Either breastfeeding will cause your extra weight to just drop off easily without your even trying, or it will cause the weight to stay stubbornly put, no matter how careful one is about watching what is eaten.

If you are breastfeeding, you'll soon discover to which group you belong. If you find you are among this second group, don't diet. Your body needs the nutrients you eat to produce the best quality milk. This is not to say that it's fine to eat a chocolate cake or a bag of cookies, but if you are eating nutritious, well-balanced meals, continue to do so. A good diet will make you feel less tired and help maintain your milk supply. Good nutrition is important at all times for good health, but it is especially important while you are nursing. If you are eating well and still maintaining a few extra pounds, don't worry about it. You will probably find that you'll lose any extra weight once your baby is weaned.

It is very difficult to regain a flat stomach once you've had a cesarean delivery. After all, the muscles have been cut through and no matter how well the muscles and tissues have been sutured back together, there is still movement during the healing process. The fact that you've stayed in shape during your pregnancy will help you to recover faster from your operation, as will the gentle exercises on the cut-out page you took with you to the hospital.

Rigorous exercises once you have your doctor's okay (usually four to six weeks after you've had your baby) will also help you to regain your figure.

Try not to be disappointed if your abdomen will never again look like it did when you were sixteen. This is just not possible after a cesarean. However, by working toward the goal of attaining your maximum physical fitness, you will be able to get back into the best shape possible.

In fact, most women's bodies change shape once they have had a child. The waistline can become slightly wider (remember poor Scarlett O'Hara), the feet slightly larger, and the breasts can become either larger or smaller. Other women become slimmer and shapelier and are happier with their postpartum bodies than before they became pregnant. There's no way to predict what changes will occur or what kind of delivery you will have, but whatever changes occur, your body can always be improved with exercise. Even a very slender body is unattractive unless it is firm and toned through proper use.

SEPARATED RECTI (ABDOMINAL) MUSCLES

Separation of the long recti muscles in the abdomen usually occurs because the abdominal muscles are weak, but it can also happen if the abdomen has been severely overstretched due to a multiple pregnancy (twins, etc.), obesity or a very large baby. Muscles in good tone are better able to bear the stress of pregnancy and childbirth, so if you have been exercising during your pregnancy this will probably not happen to you. One woman I know who had this condition hadn't exercised at all either during or between her first and second pregnancies. No wonder her poor abdominals had become weak!

Separated recti muscles can lead to fatigue and lower back pain so just to make sure this hasn't happened, check your abdomen about your third postpartum day.

Elizabeth Noble, in her book *Essential Exercises for the Childbearing Year*, recommends checking yourself this way: Lie on your back with your knees bent. Press the fingers of one hand firmly into the area around your navel. Slowly lift your head and shoulders about eight inches off the bed or floor. Is there a gap, or are your fingers pushed away by your abdominal muscles?

If one or two fingers remain in the gap, do not be alarmed. This slight tissue slackness will correct itself without special attention (although exercising wouldn't hurt). If, however, you can fit three, four, or more fingers between the tight bands of muscle, then there has been a separation that needs to be corrected.

Check with your doctor or midwife to confirm your diagnosis. If the muscles are separated, or if you just want to strengthen and flatten your abdomen anyway, start the following routine. Do not begin the regular postnatal exercise routines until the condition has been corrected.

1. Ms. Noble recommends that you lie on your back with your knees bent and your hands crossed over your abdomen. As you exhale, lift your head off the bed or floor and push the abdominal muscles toward each other in the center with your hands. Slowly lower your head and inhale. Do this about forty times a day.

2. Be particularly attentive to your posture since poor posture will weaken your abdominal muscles further. Make a con-

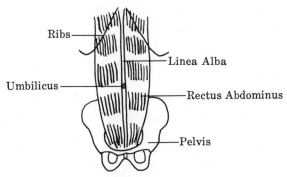

Normally, the recti muscles lie very close together.

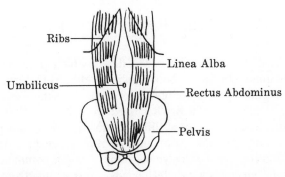

Over stretching of the recti muscles can cause them to separate.

certed effort to stand tall during the day, and to sit with a straight spine.

3. Do deep abdominal breathing fifty times a day. Relax your abdomen when you inhale, tighten and flatten your abdomen each time you exhale. Do the deep breathing while you change your baby's diaper, whenever you wash a dish or each time you listen to someone speak. It's a good habit to get into, anyway, and will help keep your abdominal muscles toned.

4. Try to move smoothly throughout the day, taking special care when you change position. To get up from your bed or the floor, roll onto your side and use your hands to push yourself up to sitting. Avoid soft chairs or couches and instead use those that can be easily gotten in and out of. Before you pick up your baby, lower the side of the crib, bend your knees, and pull your abdomen in to give your back the support it needs. (You don't need lower back problems on top of everything else right now, I'm sure.)

5. Support your abdominals when you cough or sneeze by using your hands to help hold the muscles together.

Within just a few weeks, your abdominal muscles will probably be back where they belong. Once you've gotten the go-ahead from your doctor or midwife, start the postpartum exercise routines that follow.

ONCE YOU ARE HOME

It's hard to do everything. The days fly by and you wonder where they've gone. (In fact, I hope you're reading this during your pregnancy because you probably won't have the time for a while afterward!) "I never realized what hard work it is!" "I've never had a more demanding job in my life!" "I was definitely not prepared for this!" All are common comments from new parents. An anecdote I heard at a conference this year exemplifies this common experience. The story concerns a new father who comes home from work and is pleased to find that his wife is already in her nightgown. He soon discovers, however, that rather than being a hint about going to bed early, his wife simply hadn't had the chance to get dressed yet! You may be a little more organized or have a little more help those first few weeks than the woman in the story, but you will also probably sympathize with her.

Being home with a newborn keeps a new parent busy, yet there are none of the obvious signs of work accomplished: clothes washed, letters written, bills paid, shopping done, or the house cleaned. Part of adjusting to the role of parenthood is the realization that taking care of a baby is a difficult, demanding, more than fulltime job, and that new priorities have to be established.

You have to decide what they are and their order of importance. They can change, as the situation dictates, so that the baby comes first at some times, and your life as a couple or your sanity and health as a person comes first at others.

If you have help at home, things will be a little easier. One of the nice things about infants is that they really don't care who's around as long as they can get fed, changed, and be held by someone warm and gentle. So, if your baby can be watched by someone else—your mother, mother-in-law, trusted babysitter, housekeeper, or nurse—you can be freed for a time to do something for you. What do *you* need most? A quiet time in the bathtub, a walk outside, a nap, or a visit to a friend? An hour or so without the baby is not the time to do the laundry, wash dishes, or prepare supper. Be sure to see to your personal needs as well as the baby's. One does not have to be at the expense of the other.

Exercise at this point is very important. You probably feel that you get all the exercise you need just doing household chores, but it's not the same. Running up and down a flight of stairs all day may seem like exercise, but it won't help strengthen muscles that have become stretched or weakened during pregnancy. It also won't relieve tension, get your abdominal muscles back in shape (especially if you've had a cesarean), or improve your self-image. But where to find the time?

It is understandable if setting aside a special time for exercise is not first on your list of priorities during your first few weeks at home. Until you can find the time to start the regular postpartum exercise program, use the body toning ideas I have listed below. They can be incorporated into your daily schedule, whether you're home or back at work, and at least you'll be doing something toward getting back in condition. These will not replace regular extended periods of exercise, but they will begin to get you back into condition.

Remember your good posture habits. This is the single most important daily exercise you can do for yourself. You no longer have a big belly to support, but it's still important to use your abdominal muscles when you walk or stand. Carrying your baby, whether it's in your arms or against your chest in a carrier, is hard on your back and shoulders. Your back still needs all the help and support it can get from your abdominal muscles, so keep them working (it's good for them, anyway), keep your lower back long and relaxed, and keep your head and chest light and lifted.

In fact, *use your abdominals all day long.* Pull them in when you go up stairs or wait for an elevator, pull them in each time you pick up your baby or older child and each time you put him or her down. Use them when you open the refrigerator door or talk on the phone. In this way, you'll be toning your abdominal muscles, making your work easier, and saving your back unnecessary wear and tear.

Every Few Hours Just Stop for a Moment

1. Let your body drop over toward the floor, and let your arms hang naturally. Drop your chin in toward your chest. Tighten your abdominal muscles, but relax your back and feel the stretch along the backs of your legs and along your spine. Take a deep breath, then as you exhale slowly unroll, vertebra by vertebra, up to standing. Once you're up, take another deep breath and let it out with a sigh.

2. Stretch your arms to the ceiling and look up. Reach your right arm even higher, stretching your ribs away from your waist. Now stretch your left arm higher than your right and stretch the ribs on your left side out of your waist. Keep changing sides, about ten times altogether. When you're done, reach with both arms toward the ceiling, circle them all the way to the back, squeezing your shoulder blades together, and finally

let them drop by your sides. This will be very good for getting the "kinks" out of your neck and back, toning your ribs and waist, and refreshing you.

3. Do three or four Head Circles (page 38) in each direction, and the same number of Shoulder Circles (page 46), and Arm Circles (page 70).

IX THE POSTNATAL EXERCISES

BEFORE YOU BEGIN

Even if you have returned to your prepregnancy weight you will probably find that your abdomen is still flabby or soft. The return of prepregnancy muscle tone takes time and work, but if you have been following the exercises in this book during your pregnancy, you will soon see all those months of hard work pay off.

You can usually start the postnatal exercises anywhere from two to four weeks following a vaginal delivery, or four to six weeks following an uncomplicated cesarean birth. *Check with your doctor or midwife* before starting. If at any time you notice that your lochia (bleeding) is getting redder, call your doctor or midwife. You are probably trying to do too much and you'll need to rest for a few days.

I have arranged the postnatal exercises in the same way as the prenatal ones: three routines of eight exercises each, with three optional standing exercises which can either start or end your exercise session. Again, spend about three to four weeks learning each new set of exercises, then go back and review them all.

Once all the postnatal exercises are familiar, feel free to create your own routine, using the chart that lists all the exercises according to the body part it works (page 18). Make sure your own routine includes at least one exercise from each category.

Also feel free to include any of your favorite prenatal exercises. I use many of these movements in my postnatal exercise classes; the only reason I have not included them among the postnatal routines is for variety's sake only.

The Postnatal Routines

Routine I

1. Leg Stretches II
2. Knee Cross
3. Knee Changes
4. Back Massage With Leg Stretch
5. Double Leg Lifting
6. Reverse Sit-ups
7. Shoulder Stretch
8. Full Circles in Stride

Routine II

1. Full Body Circles With Arms
2. Sitting Leg Slide
3. Leg Lowering
4. Snow Angels
5. Leg Crossovers
6. Coccyx Balance
7. Sitting Hamstring Stretch
8. Grace

Routine III

1. Side Knee Rolling
2. Double Leg Slide
3. Side Thighs
4. Shoulder Circles
5. Chest Lift
6. Leg Circles
7. Hip Circles
8. Shoulder Stand

Postnatal Standing Exercise I
Postnatal Standing Exercise II
Postnatal Standing Exercise III
A Longer Postnatal Exercise Routine

| POSTNATAL
| ROUTINE

1. Leg Stretches II

PURPOSE: To stretch, tone, and strengthen the muscles in the legs and abdomen.

TO START: Lie on your back with your knees bent and the soles of your feet on the floor, about hip width apart. Rest your arms straight down by your sides.

INHALE: Bring your left knee in toward your chest.

EXHALE: Flatten your abdomen and straighten your left leg toward the ceiling. Keep your hips and buttocks on the floor.

INHALE: Flex your left foot pressing your heel toward the ceiling. Feel the stretch along the back of your leg.

EXHALE: Tighten your abdominal muscles and slowly lower your left leg to the floor. Make sure your lower back stays flat against the floor.

TOTAL: Four times on each leg.

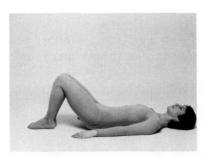

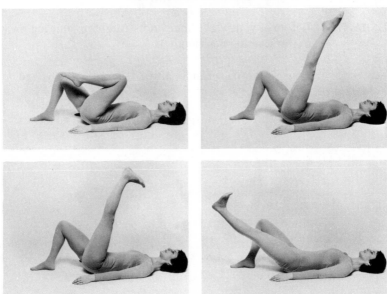

| POSTNATAL
| ROUTINE

2. Knee Cross

PURPOSE: To stretch and tone the hips, waist, and upper body.

TO START: Lie flat on the floor with your legs straight. Place your arms straight out to your sides, just below shoulder height, palms down to the floor.

INHALE: Bend your right knee in toward your chest and place your left hand on the outside of your knee.

EXHALE: Pull your right leg up and across your body to the floor and feel the stretch across your waist, back, shoulder, and arm. Keep your left leg straight.

INHALE: Roll your hips back to the floor.

EXHALE: Let go of your right knee and straighten your leg back to the starting position.

TOTAL: Four times to each side, alternating sides each time.

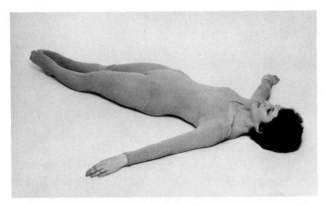

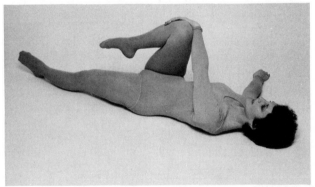

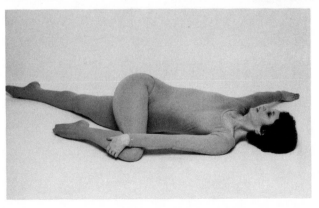

| POSTNATAL
| ROUTINE

3. Knee Changes

PURPOSE: To strengthen the abdomen.

NOTE: This exercise is totally for the abdominal muscles, even though the legs move. Don't turn it into a leg exercise. Keep your abdomen flat the whole time and do rib, rather than abdominal breathing. If the exercise is done correctly, you should feel that your legs are light, moving easily and fluidly from a strong abdomen.

TO START: Lie flat on the floor. Draw your left knee in toward your chest, placing your hands just below (not on) your left knee. Lift your right leg off the floor and feel your lower back press into the floor. If you feel any pain in the groin area, lift your right leg higher.

            Your head can either be on or off the floor, whichever you prefer. It is easier, however, to keep your lower back on the floor with your head and shoulders lifted.

INHALE deeply.

EXHALE: Change legs.

TOTAL: Ten times on each leg alternating legs each time.

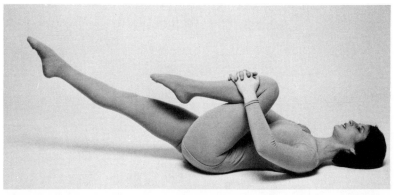

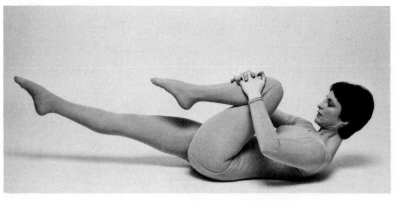

┃ POSTNATAL
┃ ROUTINE

4. Back Massage With Leg Stretch

PURPOSE: To stretch, tone, and strengthen the legs, hips, and back.

TO START: Lie on your back with your knees bent and the soles of your feet on the floor, about hip width apart.

INHALE deeply.

EXHALE: Roll your spine off the floor, vertebra by vertebra, just the way you did in the prenatal Back Massage (page 34).

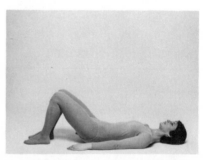

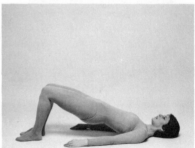

INHALE: Bend your right knee in toward your chest. Relax
            your rib cage and shoulders, but keep pressing up-
            ward underneath your buttocks and left thigh. If your
            lower back hurts, you're pushing in the wrong place!

EXHALE: Stretch your right leg straight, reaching your toes
            toward the ceiling.

INHALE: Bend your knee back in toward your chest.

EXHALE: Return your right foot to the floor.

            Repeat with your other leg. Inhale deeply, then roll
            your spine back to the floor as you exhale.

TOTAL: Three times.

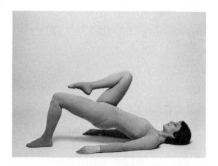

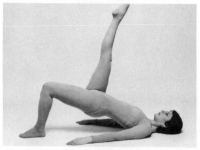

┃ POSTNATAL
┃ ROUTINE

5. Double Leg Lifting

PURPOSE: To tone the waist, hips, and legs.

TO START: Lie on your right side with your body on one straight line, resting your head on your right hand. Place your left hand in front of your chest, palm flat on the floor. Point your feet.

INHALE deeply.

EXHALE: Tighten your abdominal muscles and your buttocks, reach your legs longer, and lift both legs off the floor, to about hip height. Try to stay on your side, on the bones, and try *not* to roll back.

INHALE: Lower your legs gently, and with control, back to the floor.

TOTAL: Six times on each side.

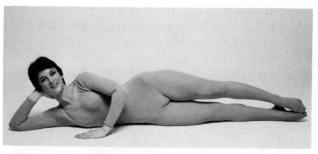

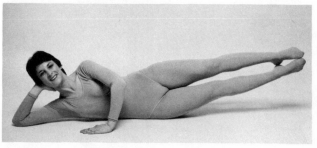

▌POSTNATAL
▌ROUTINE

6. Reverse Sit-ups

PURPOSE: To tone and strengthen the abdominal muscles.

NOTE: I rarely see Sit-ups done properly. People think they are doing them right, but they use their hands, their chins, their heads, or their shoulders to do the work their abdominals should be doing.

When you do Sit-ups, concentrate on keeping the entire front of your body flat and working—never let those muscles form big, unsightly bulges. Also try to move very smoothly and evenly as you roll your spine on and off the floor. Find the breathing pattern and tempo that works best for you.

It is not important that you roll completely to the floor. This takes a lot of abdominal strength and you may need time to build up to it. Only roll a quarter or half of the way down until you feel confident enough and strong enough to go further. Keep in mind that it's not how low you can roll, but how correctly you can move.

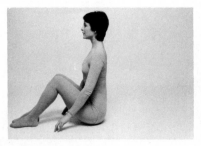 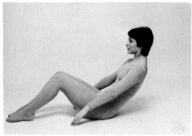

TO START: Sit tall with your knees bent and your feet placed about six inches apart. Let your fingers rest lightly on the floor by your sides.

Breathe as you roll your spine, vertebra by vertebra, to the floor. Keep your chin in toward your chest, your shoulders relaxed, and your toes on the floor. *Don't rest at the bottom.* Let your head touch the floor, bring your chin in to your chest, and roll *smoothly* up to sitting.

TOTAL: Eight times.

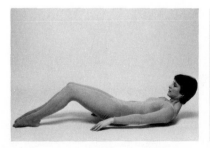
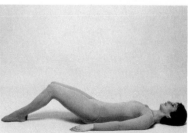

7. Shoulder Stretch

PURPOSE: To stretch and relax the muscles in the chest and upper back.

TO START: Sit tailor fashion with your legs crossed. Put your arms behind you and intertwine your fingers.

BREATHING: Breathe slowly and deeply throughout. Remain still and concentrate on relaxing during the inhalations; allow your arms to move during the exhalations only.

INHALE deeply.

Slowly stretch and lift your arms up and away from your body. When you've reached your limit, drop your chin in toward your chest and round your spine over. Stay there for a minute or so and keep lengthening your arms away from you, toward the ceiling.

To finish, slowly unroll your spine to sitting. Try not to move your arms, however. Once you are up, gently release your fingers and let your arms float out to your sides. Feel very open and wide through your back and chest. Slowly lower your arms to your sides.

TOTAL: Once.

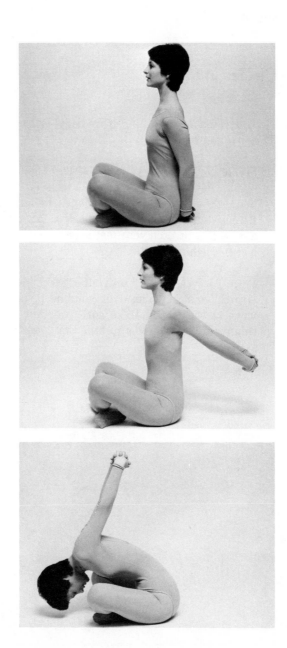

POSTNATAL ROUTINE

8. Full Circles in Stride

PURPOSE: To stretch and tone the entire body—ribs, waist, legs, and upper body.

TO START: Sit on the floor with your legs straight and *comfortably* open. Use the muscles in your back to sit very tall. (You should feel those sit bones underneath you.) Reach your arms out to your sides, just below shoulder height. Stretch your feet longer, and turn our your legs in the hip sockets.

INHALE: Place your right hand on your right ankle or calf and stretch your left arm over your head, bending sideways at the waist. Make sure your left buttock and thigh stay on the floor, and that your knees stay straight.

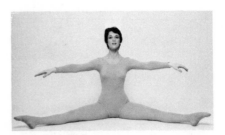

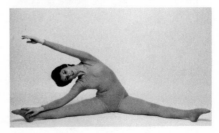

EXHALE: Circle your arms and body to the front and allow your head to relax forward. Keep your shoulders relaxed as you stretch your body out from your hips.

INHALE: Continue the circle as you place your left hand on your left ankle or calf and stretch to the left side. Keep your right leg turned out and feel the stretch run down your right side and along the inside of your right leg.

EXHALE: Tighten your abdominal muscles and roll your spine up to center.

TOTAL: Four times to each side, reversing direction each time.

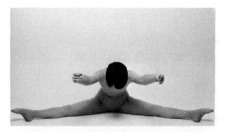

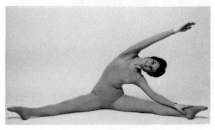

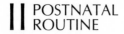 POSTNATAL
ROUTINE

1. Full Body Circles With Arms

PURPOSE: To tone the arms, waist, and upper body and to relax
             the neck and shoulders.

TO START: Sit tailor fashion with your legs crossed and your arms
             by your sides.

INHALE: Place your left hand on the floor and stretch your right
             arm over your head as you bend to the left. Think
             about pressing your right thigh toward the floor and
             your right arm in the opposite direction, making sure
             to keep both hips on the floor. Feel a long stretch
             along your right side.

EXHALE: Circle your arms and body to the front and allow your
             head to relax in toward your chest. Stretch your body
             out from your waist along your spine rather than from
             your shoulders.

INHALE: Continue the circle. Place your right hand on the floor
             and stretch your left arm to the right side. Now you
             should feel the stretch down the entire left side of your
             body.

EXHALE: Roll back to the starting position with the shoulders
             relaxed and the ribs lifted away from the hips. Feel
             very tall.

TOTAL: Six circles to each side, reversing directions each time.

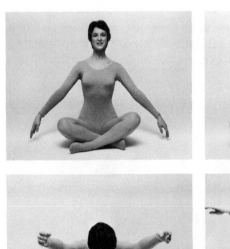
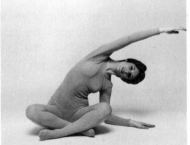
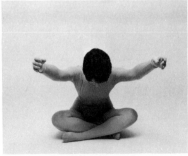
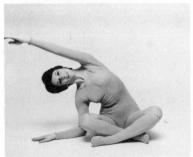

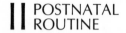

|| POSTNATAL
|| ROUTINE

2. Sitting Leg Slide

(Adapted from a Kathy Grant alignment exercise.)

PURPOSE: To strengthen the muscles in the back and abdomen.

NOTE: Your back should stay straight throughout this exercise. If you can, sit sideways to a mirror so that you can check.

TO START: Sit tall with your knees bent and the soles of your feet on the floor. Keep your knees and feet together. Your hands can either be by your sides or on your knees.

INHALE deeply.

EXHALE: Grow taller as you slide your feet away from you until your knees are straight. Think of creating a strong vertical line with your spine and a long horizontal line with your legs.

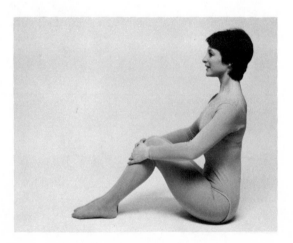

INHALE: Flex, then point your feet, but keep your back long and straight. Sit even taller.

EXHALE: Tighten your abdominals and bend your knees back toward you.

TOTAL: Six times.

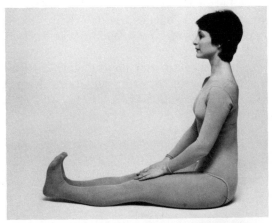

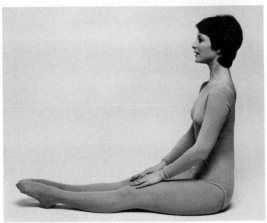

|| POSTNATAL
|| ROUTINE

3. Leg Lowering

PURPOSE: To strengthen the abdominal muscles.

NOTE: It's more important to do this exercise correctly than
              to be able to lower your legs all the way to the floor.
              It's better to be able to move your legs three inches
              with your abdominals working than to lower your legs
              three feet using (and straining) your back.

TO START: Lean back onto your elbows and forearms and bend
              your knees in toward your chest. Keep your back
              straight and your chest lifted.

INHALE: Stretch your legs toward the ceiling with your toes
              pointed.

EXHALE: Make your abdomen very flat and slowly lower your
              legs to where you can still comfortably control them
              with your abdominal muscles. Stop if you feel any pain
              in your lower back. (If you do feel pain, it probably
              means that your legs are going too low.)

INHALE: Bend your knees back in toward your chest and again
              straight up to the ceiling to repeat.

TOTAL: Eight times.

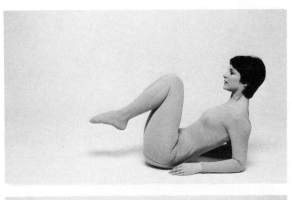

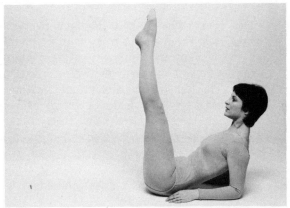

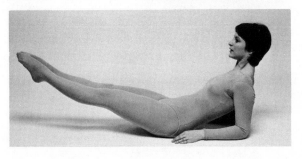

|| POSTNATAL
|| ROUTINE

4. Snow Angels

(Remember lying in the snow and moving your arms up and down to make angels' wings? That's the movement in this exercise.)

PURPOSE: To relax and stretch the muscles in the back, neck, and shoulders.

TO START: Lie flat on the floor with your knees bent and the soles of your feet on the floor. Place your arms straight down by your sides.

BREATHE slowly and naturally throughout.

Place your palms down to the floor. Slowly slide your arms along the floor out from your sides and up as far as you can toward your ears. Keep your palms and thumbs flat on the floor and let each arm describe a semicircle. Keep your arms straight, without bending at the wrist or elbow, and feel your arms moving from your shoulder blades and back. Press your shoulders down and keep your ribs and upper back flat to the floor as you move your arms higher.

Slowly slide your arms back to your sides.

Open your palms to the ceiling and keep them up, hands flat on the floor, as you repeat the half circles. Your arms will probably have greater mobility in this position and they may go higher than when the palms were down.

TOTAL: Four times in each hand position.

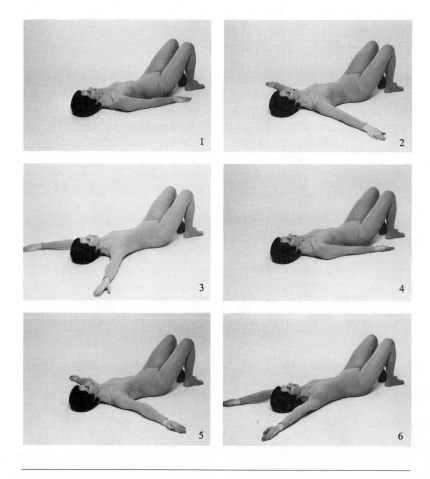

‖ POSTNATAL ROUTINE

5. Leg Crossovers

PURPOSE: To stretch and tone the muscles through the hips, waist, and legs.

TO START: Lie flat on the floor with your legs straight and your toes stretched. Place your arms straight out to the sides, just below shoulder height, palms down.

INHALE deeply.

EXHALE: Tighten your abdomen and stretch your left leg toward the ceiling, keeping it straight. *Height is not important.* Think instead about stretching both legs away from each other and of keeping your left thigh on the floor.

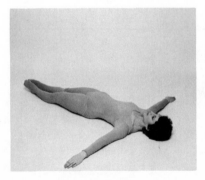
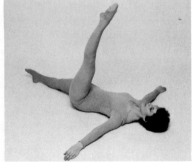

INHALE: Reach your left leg across your body to touch the floor on your right side. Allow your left hip and shoulder to lift off the floor, but try not to move your left hand.

EXHALE: Reach your left arm longer and roll your shoulder, ribs, and hip back to the floor as you stretch your left leg back toward the ceiling.

INHALE: Stretch and lower your left leg back to the floor.

TOTAL: Six times to each side, alternating legs each time.

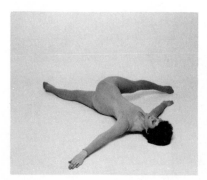
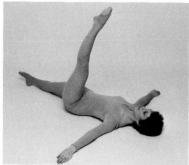

|| POSTNATAL
|| ROUTINE

6. Coccyx Balance

PURPOSE: To strengthen the abdominal and back muscles.

NOTE: This is a very difficult exercise and requires a great deal of back and abdominal strength. Be patient, mastery will come with time and practice.

TO START: Lie flat on the floor with your arms straight down by your sides.

INHALE deeply.

EXHALE: In one smooth motion, lift your body to balance on your coccyx (or tailbone). To get up, reach your hands for your toes at the same time that you bend your knees in toward your chest.

INHALE: Take hold of your ankles or calves.

EXHALE: Lift your chest and back and straighten your legs and back. (Press your body forward toward your legs, not the reverse. You'll soon discover that the tendency is to fall back.)

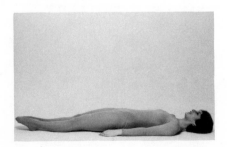

INHALE.

EXHALE: Let go of your legs, tighten your abdominals, round your lower spine, and unroll, vertebra by vertebra, back to the floor. Your head and feet should touch the floor at the same time. (If this is too difficult at first, bend your knees, place your feet on the floor, and then roll your spine to the floor, like a reverse sit-up.)

TOTAL: Four times.

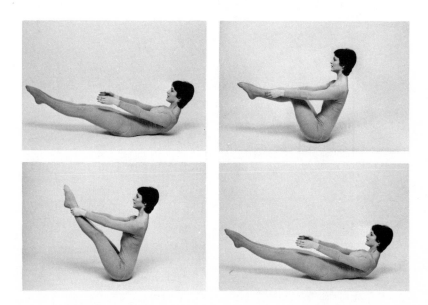

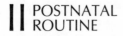

POSTNATAL
ROUTINE

7. Sitting Hamstring Stretch

PURPOSE: To stretch the muscles in the backs of the legs (the hamstring muscles).

TO START: Sit with your legs straight out in front of you. Relax your body over your legs.

INHALE: Flex your feet and reach your heels away from you. Lengthen the backs of your knees. You will probably feel most of the stretch along the backs of your legs, although you may feel your spine stretching also.

EXHALE: Point your feet and relax your body a little closer to your legs.

TOTAL: Five times.

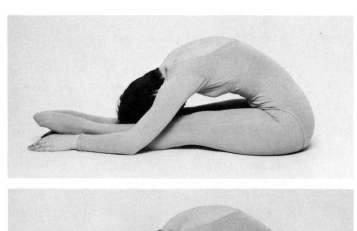

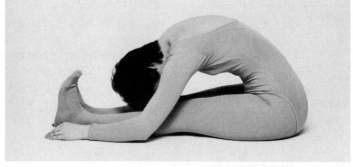

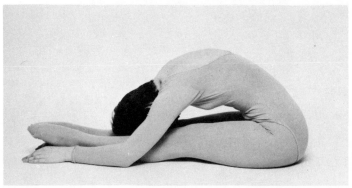

‖ POSTNATAL
‖ ROUTINE

8. Grace

PURPOSE: To tone and firm the waist, hips, thighs, and abdomen.

NOTE: This exercise should be done in one smooth motion, moving from one side to the next, and circling the arms in one easy motion.

TO START: Sit on your left hip with your feet tucked close to your right hip. Your weight will be on your left hip. Reach both arms out to the right side, in the direction of your feet.

INHALE: Stretching your arms longer to the side and then up to the ceiling, lift your hips off the floor. Your body should now be in one straight line from your knees to your hands.

EXHALE: Pull your abdomen in, continue the circle with the arms reaching now to the left side, and sit *gently* onto your right hip.

TOTAL: Ten times altogether, five to each side.

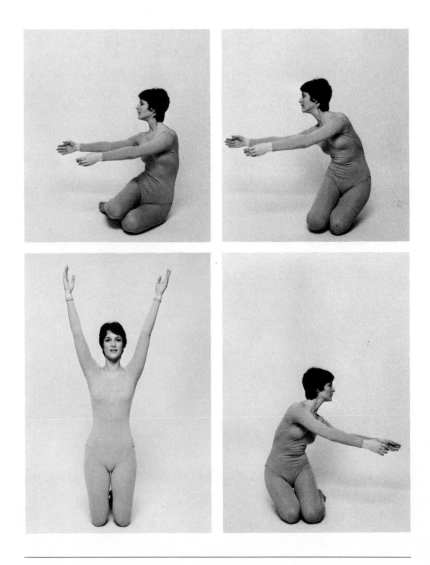

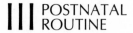

POSTNATAL ROUTINE

1. Side Knee Rolling

PURPOSE: To tone and firm the hips and waist and to relax the muscles in the lower back.

TO START: Lie on your back with both knees bent in toward your chest. Place your arms straight out to your sides just below shoulder height, with your palms down to the floor.

INHALE: Roll your knees to the floor on your left side, but try to keep your right hand and shoulder on the floor.

EXHALE: Use your abdominal muscles to roll back to center.

TOTAL: Six times to each side, alternating sides each time.

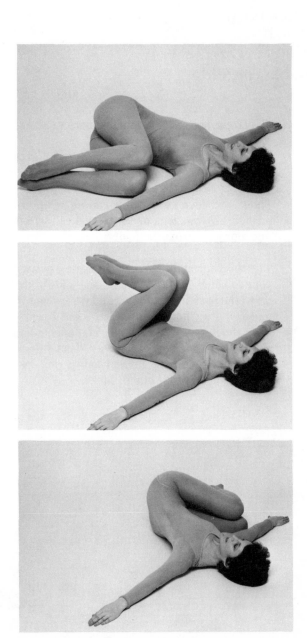

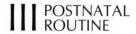 POSTNATAL
ROUTINE

2. Double Leg Slide

PURPOSE: To strengthen the abdominal muscles.

TO START: Lie on your back with your knees bent and the soles of
            your feet on the floor.

INHALE: Slide your feet away from you along the floor. Only
            straighten your legs as far as you can without releas-
            ing your back from the floor.

EXHALE: Tighten your abdominal muscles, do a pelvic tilt, press
            your lower back to the floor, and slide your feet back
            up to the starting position. Make sure your abdominal
            muscles stay flat—do not let them bulge—and that
            your shoulders stay relaxed. You may at first only be
            able to slide your legs part way. That's fine. It's more
            important to develop correct habits than to be able to
            straighten your legs out all the way.

TOTAL: Six times.

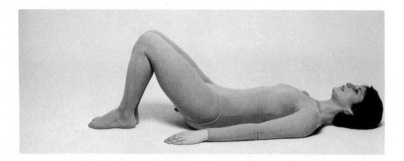

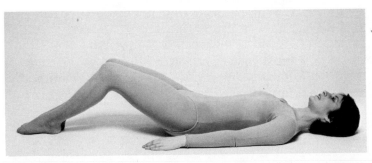

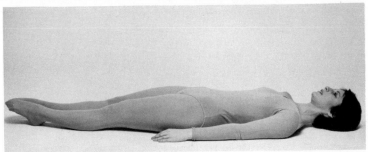

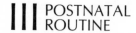

III POSTNATAL ROUTINE

3. Side Thighs

PURPOSE: To tone the inner and outer thighs.

NOTE: You may have to experiment a little to find the leg position that's best for you. To prevent your bent leg from helping to lift the straight one, you'll need to determine whether the bottom knee needs to be closer in toward you or farther away. Adjust the top leg so that you feel the work in your thigh, not in your hip.

TO START: Lie on your left side and rest your head on your left hand. Bend both knees in toward your chest. Straighten the top leg out so it's at about a forty-five degree angle to your body. Flex your right foot.

INHALE deeply.

EXHALE: Stretch your right heel away from you, flexing your foot more strongly, and stretch your leg off the floor, to about hip height.

INHALE: Lower your leg gently and with control back to the floor.

TOTAL: Ten times on each leg.

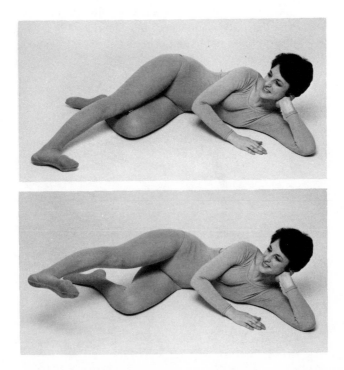

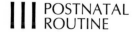 POSTNATAL
ROUTINE

4. Shoulder Circles

PURPOSE: To relax and stretch the upper back, neck, and shoulder areas.

TO START: Sit tailor fashion with your legs crossed. Rest your hands on your knees.

BREATHE slowly and naturally throughout.

Slowly roll your shoulders in a circle, drawing them forward and feeling your shoulder blades open and your back widen, lifting them up in a shrug, rolling them to the back and squeezing your shoulder blades together in the back, and then relaxing them into their natural position.

TOTAL: Eight circles in each direction.

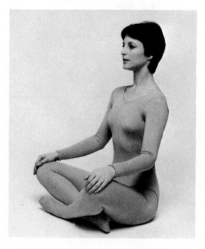
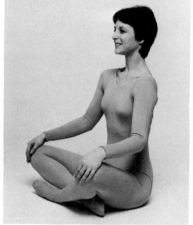

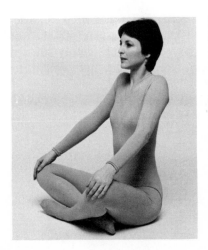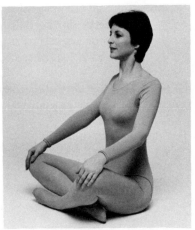

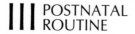 POSTNATAL ROUTINE

5. Chest Lift

PURPOSE: To strengthen the muscles in the back and chest and to stretch the muscles in the backs of the legs.

NOTE: This is very good for those women with rounded shoulders, a very common problem with a newborn around. They get that way from all that cuddling, feeding, and carrying (especially in infant carries worn on the chest).

TO START: Sit with your legs straight out in front of you. Relax your body over, with your head toward your knees.

INHALE.

EXHALE: Flatten your abdomen, slide your arms behind you, and roll your spine down to the floor, vertebra by vertebra. Keep your chin in toward your chest as you roll to the floor, and use your hands for support.

INHALE: Lift your chest to the ceiling as if you were a marionette or rag doll being pulled by a ring attached to your breastbone. Keep your neck absolutely relaxed and let your head hang back as you lift up to sitting.

EXHALE: Continue all the way up, let your head drop forward, and relax your body over your legs.

TOTAL: Six times.

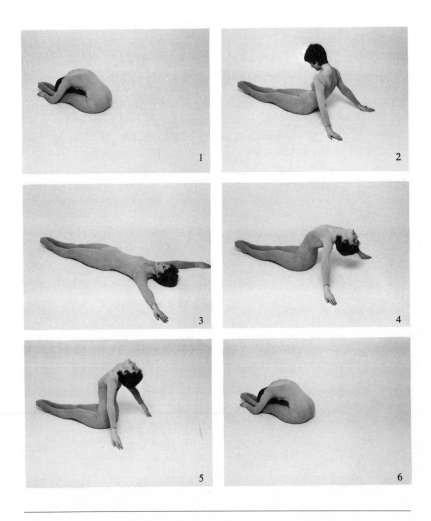

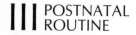

POSTNATAL
ROUTINE

6. Leg Circles

PURPOSE: To tone and firm the legs and abdomen.

TO START: Lie on the floor with your legs straight and your arms
            straight out to your sides, just below shoulder height.

INHALE: Lift and stretch your left leg toward the ceiling. Stretch
            and lengthen your right leg at the same time.

EXHALE: Flex your left foot, turn out your left leg, and circle
            your left leg out to your left side and back down to the
            starting position. Make sure both hips stay on the floor
            the entire time.

INHALE: Reverse the circle. Lift your left leg off the floor and
            swing it out to your left side. Keep your toes pointed.

EXHALE: Tighten your abdominal muscles and use them to lift
            your leg up to the ceiling and to lower your leg straight
            out and down to the floor.

TOTAL: Four times on each leg.

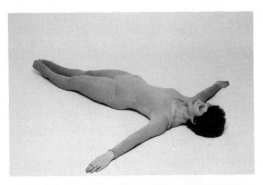

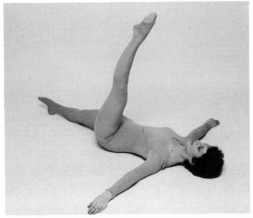

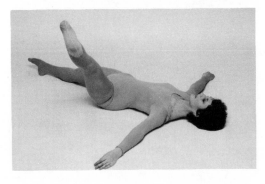

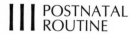 POSTNATAL
ROUTINE

7. Hip Circles

PURPOSE: To tone the hips, waist, and legs.

NOTE: This should be performed in one smooth motion as
             your hips describe a wide circle in the air. Find the
             momentum from the initial thrust through the hips to
             get you up and over the top, then roll smoothly back to
             the floor to complete the circle.

TO START: Lie on your back with your knees bent and the soles of
             your feet on the floor. Do the Back Massage from the
             prenatal exercises (page 34) three to four times to
             warm up your back. Place your arms out to the sides
             just below shoulder height, palms down.

INHALE deeply.

EXHALE: Roll your knees to the right and tighten your buttocks
             and the backs of your thighs, exactly like you did in
             the prenatal exercise, the Side Press (page 46). Use
             the side momentum to lift your hips off the floor and up
             toward the ceiling.

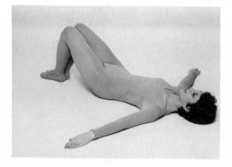

INHALE: Continue the circle to the left and touch your left side to the floor when you come down. Relax to the starting position before reversing direction.

TOTAL: Four times to each direction, alternating sides each time.

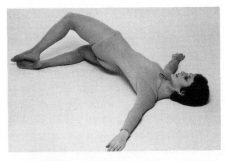

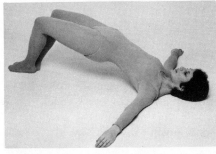

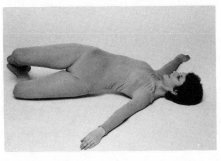

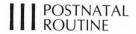 POSTNATAL
ROUTINE

8. Shoulder Stand

PURPOSE: For the entire body—hips, waist, legs, and back.

NOTE: You may want to put a flat pillow or towel under your head and neck for comfort.

There may be some soreness in your neck and back after this exercise. That's because we're not used to supporting our body weight with our neck and shoulders, and because in this exercise, the weight of the body is used to stretch the back and legs. Do not do this exercise if you have back problems such as scoliosis or lordosis of the spine, or disc problems.

BREATHE naturally throughout the starting movements.

TO START: Lie on your back with your arms by your sides and your knees in toward your chest. Roll your knees back over your head so that your knees rest by your ears. Your feet do not have to touch the floor. If you have trouble getting into this position, start from sitting and then roll back.

INHALE: Relax your shoulders into the floor.

EXHALE: Flatten your abdomen and slowly straighten your legs behind you. Again, don't be concerned if your feet don't touch the floor—the stretch will come with time and practice. Feel the stretch along your spine and the backs of your legs. Bend and straighten your legs three-four times.

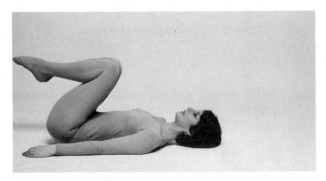

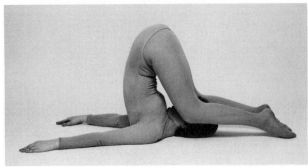

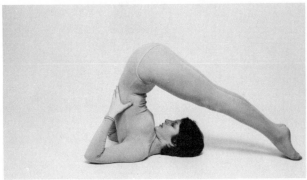

Continued

INHALE: Place your hands on your waist.

EXHALE: Flatten your abdomen and lift both legs to the ceiling.
           Lift your hips out of your waist and stretch your legs
           up toward the ceiling, toes pointed.

INHALE deeply.

EXHALE: Slowly lower your legs to the floor behind your head.
           Raise and lower your legs three to four times.

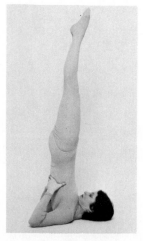

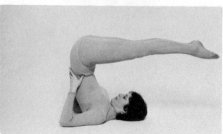

To Roll
Down:

Bend your knees back toward your shoulders. Press your thighs in toward your chest and your hands into the floor by your sides. Roll your spine back to the floor, vertebra by vertebra, until your entire back is on the floor.

Rest for a minute or so and breathe deeply and slowly. Sit up and do some slow Head Circles (page 38) or Body Circles (page 48) to relax your neck and upper back.

Total: Once.

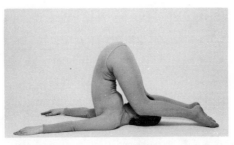

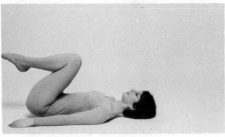

| POSTNATAL
| STANDING EXERCISE

Pliés/Relevés II

PURPOSE: To tone the entire body, but especially the legs and inner thighs.

TO START: Stand with your feet comfortably open and your toes facing outward, arms comfortably down at your sides, or on your hips.

BREATHE naturally throughout.

Slowly bend your knees open just the way you did in the prenatal Pliés (page 76). Press your heels off the floor into relevé and balance on the balls and toes of your feet.

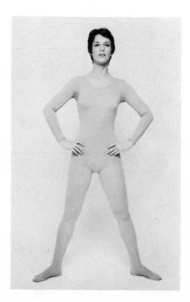
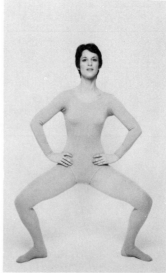

Slowly straighten your legs. Keep lifting your heels higher off the floor toward your calves. Your legs should feel strong (they are your support, like columns in a building), but allow your body to be light. Use your abdominals to maintain good posture, and to help you balance over your feet.

Stay tall as you slowly (and with control from your inner thighs and abdominals) lower your heels to the floor.

TO REVERSE THE MOVEMENT:

Keep your legs straight as you lift your heels off the floor into relevé. Keep them high as you bend your knees open, slowly lower your heels to the floor, and then slowly straighten your legs once more.

TOTAL: Four times.

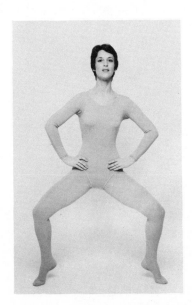
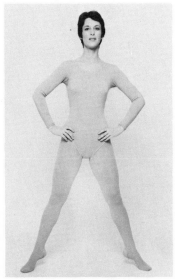

11 POSTNATAL STANDING EXERCISE

Table Top II

PURPOSE: To stretch and tone the entire body.

TO START: Stand with your feet parallel and about hip width apart.

INHALE: Stretch your arms to the ceiling (but leave your shoulders down).

EXHALE: Stretch your body forward from the hips (like a "Barbie" doll) until your back is parallel to the floor like a table top. Keep your neck and arms in line with the rest of your spine.

INHALE.

EXHALE: Let your back round and drop your arms and head toward the floor.

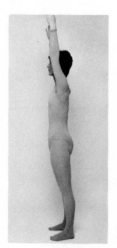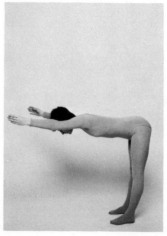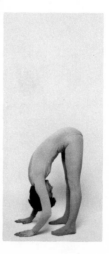

INHALE: Bend your knees, round your spine more, and put your head on your knees and your hands on the floor.

EXHALE: *Try* to leave your hands and body where they are and slowly straighten your legs completely. You should feel the stretch along the backs of your legs.

INHALE: Relax your body completely and let your arms and head hang.

EXHALE: Tighten your abdominals and unroll your spine, vertebra by vertebra, to standing.

TOTAL: Four times.

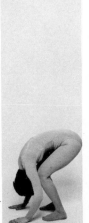
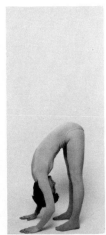
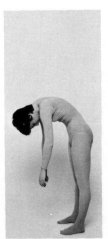
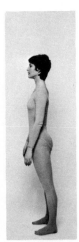

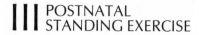

III POSTNATAL STANDING EXERCISE

Standing Side Stretch II

PURPOSE: To stretch and tone the entire body.

TO START: Stand with your legs comfortably apart, your toes fac-
            ing outward. Reach your arms straight out to your
            sides, palms down.

INHALE: Bend your left knee. Bend your right arm and your
            body over to the left. Reach both arms to the left,
            feeling the stretch along your right side.

EXHALE: Keep your left knee bent, but straighten your body
            and arms back to center.

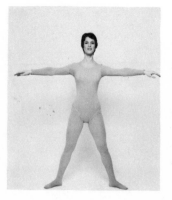 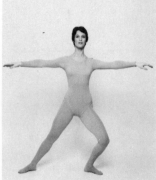

INHALE: Stretch to the right side. Relax your left ankle and
             bend your left knee even more. Feel a long stretch
             along your left side.

EXHALE: Tighten your abdominal muscles, press your left heel
             into the floor, and straighten your left knee using the
             inner thigh muscles in your left leg. You should now
             be back in the starting position.

TOTAL: Three times to each side, reversing the bent knee each
             time.

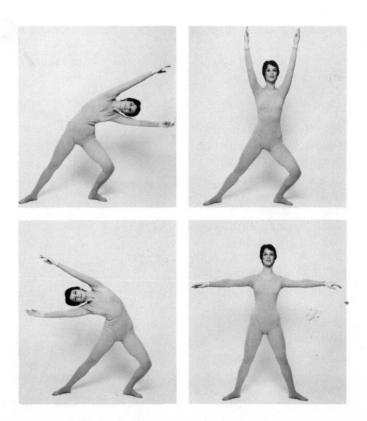

A LONGER POSTNATAL EXERCISE ROUTINE

If you would like to exercise for an hour instead of the fifteen or twenty minutes each that the suggested routine takes, try doing all of the postnatal exercises in the following order. They are arranged so that you will begin with the simpler and easier movements and progress to those that are more strenuous, warming the muscles gradually.

They are also arranged so that different parts of your body will be worked on successive exercises, alternating exercises for the legs, arms, hips, waist, abdomen and upper body. You will also be alternating sitting exercises with the ones when you are on your back and side so that you do not remain in any one position for an extended period of time.

Feel free to include or substitute any exercises from the prenatal programs into this routine.

1. Leg Stretches II (pg 108)
2. Double Leg Slide (pg 142)
3. Snow Angels (pg 130)
4. Side Knee Rolling (pg 140)
5. Knee Cross (pg 110)
6. Knee Changes (pg 112)
7. Back Massage With Leg Stretch (pg 114)
8. Side Thighs (pg 144)
9. Full Body Circles With Arms (pg 124)
10. Sitting Leg Slide (pg 126)
11. Shoulder Stretch (pg. 120)
12. Leg Lowering (pg 128)
13. Shoulder Circles (pg 146)
14. Reverse Sit-ups (pg 118)

15. Grace (pg 138)
16. Leg Crossovers (pg 132)
17. Hip Circles (pg 152)
18. Leg Circles (pg 150)
19. Shoulder Stand (pg 154)
20. Coccyx Balance (pg 134)
21. Sitting Hamstring Stretch (pg 136)
22. Chest Lift (pg 148)
23. Double Leg Lifting (pg 116)
24. Full Circles in Stride (pg 122)
25. Pliés/Relevés II (pg 158)
26. Standing Side Stretch II (pg 162)
27. Table Top II (pg 160)